SURVIVING CANCER AS A FAMILY

AND HELPING
CO-SURVIVORS THRIVE

Board of Advisors

SURVIVING CANCER AS A FAMILY

AND HELPING CO-SURVIVORS THRIVE

Catherine A. Marshall
Editor

Foreword by
Elizabeth Kendall

Disability Insights and Issues
Catherine A. Marshall and Elizabeth Kendall, Series Editors

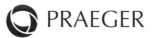 PRAEGER

AN IMPRINT OF ABC-CLIO, LLC
Santa Barbara, California • Denver, Colorado • Oxford, England

Library of Congress Cataloging-in-Publication Data

Surviving cancer as a family and helping co-survivors thrive / Catherine A. Marshall, editor ; foreword by Elizabeth Kendall.
   p.cm.—(Disability insights and issues)
  Includes bibliographical references and index.
  ISBN 978-0-313-37894-2 (hardcopy : alk. paper)—ISBN 978-0-313-37895-9 (ebook)
   1. Cancer—Psychological aspects. 2. Cancer—Patients—Family relationships. 3. Children of cancer patients. I. Marshall, Catherine A. II. Series: Disability insights and issues. [DNLM: 1. Neoplasms—psychology. 2. Caregivers—psychology. 3. Family—psychology. 4. Family Health. 5. Family Relations. 6. Survivors—psychology. QZ 200 S9637 2010]
  RC262.S865 2010
  616.99′4–dc22   2010004106

ISBN: 978-0-313-37894-2
EISBN: 978-0-313-37895-9

14 13 12 11 10   1 2 3 4 5

This book is also available on the World Wide Web as an eBook.
Visit www.abc-clio.com for details.

Praeger
An Imprint of ABC-CLIO, LLC

ABC-CLIO, LLC
130 Cremona Drive, P.O. Box 1911
Santa Barbara, California 93116-1911

This book is printed on acid-free paper ∞

Manufactured in the United States of America

Copyright Acknowledgment

Excerpts from Catherine A. Marshall, 'Family and Culture: Using Autoethnography to Inform Rehabilitation Practice with Cancer Survivors.' *Journal of Applied Rehabilitation Counseling*, 39, no. 1 (2008), 9–19. Reprinted with permission of the National Rehabilitation Counseling Association.

CONTENTS

Disability is often viewed as a negative event, but what about those who thrive and flourish despite their disability? This new series is based on stories of people with disabilities and their families coping and, indeed, thriving. Readers will learn from these stories, as well as from professionals and researchers, about how best to live with and manage their disability—how to use resources in the environment, how to find peer support, and how to be in control of their treatment and service options. The series will explore the role of personal, social, and environmental supports in the process of adjusting to and managing life with a disability.

How can interventions focus on coping and thriving, rather than problems and deficits? This series will explore, for instance, what we know about strengths-based interventions, consumer-driven approaches to service delivery, and the role of creativity in coping. Juxtaposing the personal views of people with disabilities, academic evidence, and practice knowledge, we show how people with disabilities participate fully in their own lives and how they and their family members can be supported in ways that assist them in building and using resources for a positive future.

This series of authored and edited books will give readers insight into the challenges, rewards, dilemmas, and solutions facing millions of people with disabilities—disabilities developed prior to or during birth, from accident or illness, and, significant now for our population, those associated with the aging process. Disabilities addressed will include, for instance, substantial hearing or visual impairment, osteoporosis, and paralysis, as well as HIV infection, AIDS, cancer, specific learning disabilities, autism, and mobility impairments. "Hidden" disabilities such as mental illness, brain injury, chronic pain, and chronic fatigue, all of which can cause considerable misunderstanding and suffering, will also be addressed.

Series Editors
Catherine A. Marshall
Elizabeth Kendall

Cancer is now widely recognized as a phenomenon that is experienced by the entire family, not just by the individual who has been diagnosed with the disease (Kristjanson & Ashcroft, 2006). Around the world, there is an ever-increasing population of families who are living with a history of cancer. Whereas the primary concern has always been diagnosis, treatment, and survival, it is now increasingly important to also attend to quality of life and long-term happiness for this entire group of people (Stanton, 2006).

Although survival rates continue to increase, little is known about the quality of life for the families of people surviving cancer. The period after treatment has ended remains relatively unexplored by anyone other than those whose lives it directly affects (Mellon, Northouse, & Weiss, 2006). For this reason, this volume is vitally important. The stories of *all* those affected by cancer are here—survivors, parents, spouses and partners, children, siblings, grandchildren, and friends.

When cancer comes into the home, its impact radiates rapidly. Cancer has a life-changing impact on every family member's views, behaviors, values, or beliefs. Interestingly, cancer survivors tend to report significantly higher levels of quality of life, less fear of cancer recurrence, and more sense of support than their family members. Ironically, though, research (Mellon et al., 2006) has shown that the best predictors of this quality of life are lower levels of family stress and high levels of social support (usually provided by family members or close friends). In contrast, the best predictors of family member quality of life are fear of recurrence and lack of social support. Thus, quality of life for those with cancer and quality of life for their family members are inextricably linked to each other, and often locked in a negative cycle of depletion.

Despite this powerful impact, family members have been found to cope well following diagnosis of cancer in their family (Pitceathly & Maguire, 2004). For some family members, however, cancer has more serious and potentially long-term consequences. Thomas, Morris, and Harman (2002) documented two types of stress experienced by family members, namely the demands of caring physically and the demands of managing emotions. Although the physical demands of cancer on a family vary with the stage of the disease and the family circumstances, a significant increase in the number and difficulty of practical tasks is always demanded of family members. Many family members express the need for help with these practical tasks and with the personal impact of this caring role. Caress, Chalmers, and Luker (2009) found that little is actually known about the practical knowledge and support family members require to provide physical care in the home. This lack of knowledge highlights the fact that families are often overlooked in the process of treating cancer.

By far the greatest demand on family members, however, is likely to be the "emotional work" associated with cancer. Family members may believe they should be "strong" and "positive," "carrying on as normal." Alternatively, they may not know how to react to the diagnosis, either withdrawing emotionally or reacting destructively. Managing their powerful and overwhelming emotions is likely to be exhausting, particularly when combined with physical exhaustion caused by disrupted routines, additional time demands, and extra roles.

These physical and emotional aspects of cancer cannot be ignored. They exist and they must be managed by family members. A corollary of these demands is that family members are often automatically labeled "caregivers" once a relative has cancer. For most family members, this label holds no sense of meaning. They just do whatever they have to do in order to manage the situation—they live from day to day, managing practical and emotional challenges as they arise, informing themselves and making decisions. It is an artificial and sometimes offensive shift that is imposed on family members, forcing them into the role of a carer simply because a family member has become ill. The authors in this volume rarely use the word *carer*. However, there is no doubt that partners and family members are critical sources of support for people who have been diagnosed with cancer. Indeed, family "caregivers" are considered to be the bedrock of care in the United States (Northouse, 2005). They provide unquantifiable amounts of unpaid and invisible support, often saving the health system enormous amounts of money. Yet the support provided to them is minimal—they are often invisible, their stress and trauma hidden and/or disregarded.

So what can be done to assist families? Although some research has suggested that family members who participate in interventions designed for "caregivers" derive only limited psychological benefits

(Pitceathly & Maguire, 2004), there is also evidence that supportive psychosocial or educational interventions can have a positive effect on family functioning following cancer (Northouse, 2005). However, other research has shown that only a small number of distressed family members consult a doctor or seek assistance for themselves. Indeed, in one study, nearly half of the partners/spouses with diagnosed emotional disorders did not receive any treatment (Haddad, Pitceathly, Jones, & Maguire, 1996).

Why, given the evidence that interventions may be helpful, do family members fail to take advantage of interventions designed to help them? A possible answer lies in the fact that standardized and traditional approaches to intervention do not suit everyone and, depending on the complex circumstances of the family, may actually interfere with their beliefs about what needs to be done at that time. For instance, four major issues have been identified as being critical to the impact of cancer on a family, and thus shed some light on the way in which interventions may need to be reviewed. Each issue must be considered carefully and understood fully to appreciate the way in which individual families manage cancer. The four issues include (1) the developmental stage and type of family, (2) the cancer illness trajectory, (3) the family responses to cancer, and (4) the behaviors of health care providers (Kristjanson & Ashcroft, 2006). Each of these issues has emerged strongly in the stories contained in this volume, demonstrating their importance to the overall experience of cancer.

There is ample evidence that these factors are important to the design of interventions. Chapters in this volume describe how the impact of the family structure and developmental stage interact with the cancer trajectory to produce different responses, and outline the importance of cultural factors in how families react to cancer. In some cultures, for instance, it may be acceptable, and even necessary, that a disease becomes public (so families can seek support, financial assistance, and treatment), but in other cultures, such public exposure can bring dismay, humiliation, and embarrassment.

Different family members may react in different ways at different times during the cancer journey—chapters in this volume demonstrate the diverse ways in which individuals have coped with and responded to cancer. Emotional distress among family members has been found to be highest between one and two years after cancer diagnosis (Haddad et al., 1996), significantly later than the timing found among those with cancer. Given that intervention systems are designed around the person with cancer, with high intensity contact in the early stages following diagnosis, there is less likelihood that the distress of families will be noticed.

The importance of the behavior of health professionals—the resources and information they deliver, the way in which they deliver treatment, and their responsiveness to families—cannot be underestimated. However, this aspect of the cancer journey is one of the least controllable features of the experience. Many families feel helpless in the presence of health professionals, whereas others have relayed stories of support and sensitivity that have altered their journey in positive ways. Chapters in this volume describe the benefit of taking control of cancer, drawing on personal strengths, finding support, and making active decisions about treatment.

People with cancer and their families appreciate when health professionals (Hagerty, Butow, Ellis, Dimitry, and Tattersall, 2005):

* Use a mix of positive and negative language in framing information;
* Summarize and check their understanding of information;
* Explain technical terms and provide an opportunity to ask questions;
* Use supportive behaviors such as listening to fears and concerns;
* Convey significant news in person and in a private, comfortable setting;
* Ensure that family members are present, particularly at significant discussions;
* Allow enough time for discussion and ensure it is free of interruptions;
* Provide emotional support and show understanding of psychosocial concerns;
* Convey honesty, a sense of trust, and hope when communicating; and
* If necessary, communicate clearly about end-of-life options to alleviate uncertainty.

In contrast to these points, decreasing hope was associated with the perception of poor communication, a pessimistic attitude, and an impersonal context. Gysels, Richardson, and Higginson (2004) found that communication training could improve the performance of health professionals in cancer care. However, without positive attitudes and beliefs based on a sound understanding of families and how they might respond to cancer, these new skills were not maintained in clinical practice over time.

This volume contains stories from many different types of people in many different types of situations, representing the uniquely personal experience of cancer—unique to each person, unique to each family, and unique to each family member. Still, commonalities are present following a cancer diagnosis: difficult early days marked by confusion, disbelief, avoidance, distress, and fear; multiple and diverse ways of coping; changes in family roles, feelings both of helplessness and of strength. It is through acknowledging our uniqueness and embracing our commonalities that we can survive cancer and thrive as families and as communities.

References

Caress, A., Chalmers, K., & Luker, K. (2009). A narrative review of interventions to support family carers who provide physical care to family members with cancer. *International Journal of Nursing Studies, 46*, 1516–1527.

Gysels, M., Richardson, A., & Higginson, I. (2004). Communication training for health professionals who care for patients with cancer: A systematic review of effectiveness. *Supportive Care in Cancer, 12*, 692–700.

Haddad, P., Pitceathly, C., Jones, B., & Maguire, P. (1996). Affective disorders in the partners of cancer patients: Prevalence, course & risk factors. *European Psychiatry, 11*, 272s–273s.

Hagerty, R., Butow, P., Ellis, M., Dimitry, S., & Tattersall, M. (2005). Communicating prognosis in cancer care: A systematic review of the literature. *Annals of Oncology, 16*, 1005–1053.

Kristjanson, L., & Ashcroft, T. (2006). The family's cancer journey: A literature review. *Journal of Clinical Oncology, 24*, 5132–5137.

Mellon, S., Northouse, L., & Weiss, L. (2006). A population-based study of the quality of life of cancer survivors and their family caregivers. *Cancer Nursing, 29*, 120–131.

Northouse, L. (2005). Helping families of patients with cancer. *Oncology Nursing Society, 32*, 743–750.

Pitceathly, C., & Maguire, P. (2004). The psychological impact of cancer on patients' partners and other key relatives: A review. *European Journal of Cancer, 39*(11), 1517–1524.

Stanton, A. (2006). Psychosocial concerns and interventions for cancer survivors. *Journal of Clinical Oncology, 24*, 5132–5137.

Thomas, C., Morris, S., & Harman, J. (2002). Companions through cancer: The care given by informal carers in cancer contexts. *Social Science & Medicine, 54*, 529–544

Elizabeth Kendall, Ph.D., Series Co-editor, *Disability Insights and Issues*
Research Professor, Griffith Institute of Health and Medical Research, Griffith University, and Associate Director of the Centre for National Research on Disability and Rehabilitation, at Griffith University

When Cancer Comes Home: Family Matters
Catherine A. Marshall

> When I was a child, books saved me from an otherwise nearly unbearable situation. I think there are many of us for whom that is the case, and we never forget the importance of books.[1]
>
> Richard Shelton
> *Crossing the Yard: Thirty Years as a Prison Volunteer*

I did not grow up in a prison, but at times, Chattanooga Valley felt like one. I left Southern Appalachia as soon as I could—first to Boston and then to Tucson—where I have pretty much remained. One day, my father was diagnosed with prostate cancer (Marshall, 2008). While I had obtained a Ph.D. from the University of Arizona and was considered by at least some of my teachers to be "smart," I knew nothing about cancer and I knew nothing about how to help my father. I did not even know exactly what he had. What was prostate cancer? What was cancer? I knew only that I did not want my father to die. When I first called my father's diagnosing physician, a urologist, I told him simply, "I do not want my father to die—of anything—ever. So what is this prostate cancer? What does he have? What needs to be done? What can I do?" I didn't feel smart. I felt scared. Over time, I had learned from my father that Southern Appalachia is a beautiful place. Our mountains protect

---

[1]Shelton, R. (2007). Tucson: The University of Arizona Press (p. 208).

us—our cultural values also protect and sustain us. I needed to help him after he was diagnosed with cancer, but I didn't know how.

Many of us have been affected personally by cancer. Written in a user-friendly way, this book provides families with 1) research- and experience-based information about how they can best understand cancer and help loved ones diagnosed with the disease, as well as 2) assist co-survivors in finding the support they need for their own distress. Family members of individuals diagnosed with cancer are, themselves, cancer survivors (*A National Action Plan*, 2004). While the impact of a cancer diagnosis on the lives of family members is recognized—affected family members are referred to as *co-survivors* of cancer—they are too often left outside of formal, readily available services and cancer treatment systems that could provide them with needed information and support.

The term "family" is used broadly in the literature and may refer to a close relative, a spouse, a life partner, or a primary caregiver/support person, among others. For instance, Gilgun (1992) noted that in addition to legal and biological factors that define family, persons define themselves as members of families, demonstrate commitment, and share a personal history. Understanding exactly how family is affected by cancer—those assuming caretaking roles and those not, and the broader systems in which they experience cancer and caretaking—is explored in this book through both research and personal experience. Influences such as culture and socioeconomic status that impact the family system within which a cancer patient is cared for are addressed.

Cancer is now shifting from being seen as a life-threatening disease that can be cured (or not) to being viewed as a chronic illness that may also result in disability (Hanson & Kriescher, 2006; Hewitt, Greenfield, & Stovall, 2005; Verbeek & Spelten, 2007; see also http://www.disability rightslegalcenter.org/about/cancerlegalresource.cfm). Pransky (2009) is only one of many chronic disease specialists to acknowledge that "cancer is also an illness that involves the entire family" (p. viii)—including the fact that the work of family members may be interrupted by cancer—and family members may benefit from disability-related resources and protections.

When work is affected, or when cancer results in disability, there are resources that can help (Chan, da Silva Cardoso, Copeland, Jones, & Fraser, 2009; Chan et al., 2008). Pransky noted that "many disability compensation systems still operate on an *antiquated assumption* that a cancer diagnosis is equivalent to permanent and total disability" (p. viii, emphasis added). We hope survivors and co-survivors will think of disability status as providing resources and protection, when needed—for instance, in the workplace. Indeed, disability resulting from cancer or its treatment may or may not be permanent (Stager, 2009); http://cancer andcareers.org/women/paperwork/filing_disability [Even though the URL includes "women," this Web site is good for men as well.]).

As co-survivors of cancer, family members will find in this book the information they need to better understand and cope with cancer in the family, thereby helping their loved one, and themselves, most effectively—yes, themselves as well! Authors who have contributed their work to chapters in this book know that family members need support (Power, 1995), often more so than their loved one with cancer (Sutherland, Dpsych, White, Jefford, & Hegarty, 2008). But there is no reason to "take sides" in the fight against and in the struggle to understand cancer. Cancer affects all of us, and family is who we are.

Kelly Corrigan (2008), a young mother fighting breast cancer while also helping to manage her father's bladder cancer, wrote, "And that's what this whole thing is about. Calling home. Instinctively. . . . There you are, clutching the phone and thanking God that you're still somebody's daughter" (p. 5). Describing her Internet searches for information to help her father, she wrote, "It's like I'm driving and I'm lost but instead of slowing down, I am gunning it—hunched over the wheel, squinting at street signs, turning impulsively" (p. 128); all this because "nothing and nobody is going to take my father away from me" (p. 117).

We fear cancer because we fear death—whatever the cause. The good news is that people survive cancer. We all know people who have survived cancer. This book contains chapters written by people who have survived cancer. Yet cancer is an "in-your-face" reminder that your loved one will die—even if not from cancer—and so we fear cancer in large part because it brings to our attention that we will lose a loved one—and we aren't ready.

> Daddy: "My pappy knew the date and time of his death."
> Me: "How's that?"
> Daddy: "The warden told him."

We would laugh! Every few years, each time my father told this joke, we would laugh. He was a joker! He survived prostate cancer for two and a half years after his diagnosis—not always joking, but certainly living with hope. He advised (Marshall, 2008),

> There is no Marcus Welby to watch out for you and make decisions in your best interests—if he's still alive, I don't know where he is or how to contact him. You really need a physician or advocate such as Lance Armstrong described in his book, *It's Not About the Bike*. The physician from Nashville's Vanderbilt University took a personal interest in Armstrong's case and advised him, first through a letter and then through phone calls, where to look for treatment and how best to pursue the treatment options. In my case, not one, not two, but three [local] doctors threw up their hands and said, "I don't know what to do—I've done all I can do. Go find yourself another doctor."

Family members must get involved in finding treatment options. Thanks to a family member connected to a university, she was able to get [me] an appointment with one of the leading oncologists in the area of prostate cancer. If you do not have such a person in your immediate family, I would suggest maybe someone in a church club, or a work associate, and see if they have a friend or family member that has had such misfortune to befall them and see who they would recommend as a prospect to advise you as to who would be the best person to assist you. Even if seeking out a support group is not what you'd ever want to do, in fact, finding a support group such as US TOO that specializes in your illness is important. I would recommend highly to at least sit in on some basic meetings. That way you would at least get some idea who the leading practitioners in the area are and you can then follow up. And most of all, regardless of your age or health, never give up! (p. 12)[2]

My father's life journey after his cancer diagnosis was much shorter than we would have liked, but together we did learn much about cancer:

* Cancer is cells that are growing out of control.
* Cancer takes the form of many different diseases.
* The cancer your loved one has may progress very differently than that of someone else with the same diagnosis.
* Cancer is life changing.
* Cancer treatment can be very expensive.
* Cancer treatment may be different for individuals with the same diagnosis.
* Doctors may give options for treatment, but leave treatment decisions to the survivor.
* The cancer experience can result in positive outcomes.

Regarding the latter, cancer provides us an opportunity to develop "peaks" in our lives as we confront the possibility of the death of our loved one—as we confront cancer as a chronic illness—or as we participate in a fight that leaves our loved one cancer free. Johnson (2009) tells us that "peaks are moments when you appreciate what you have . . ." (p. 24). Cancer, by anyone's definition, is a "valley," yet Johnson advises that "you change your valley into a peak when you find and use the good that is hidden in the bad time . . ." (p. 31). Importantly, and in line with the purpose of this book, "a personal peak is a triumph over fear" (p. 68). It is hard to think of personal peaks when trying to understand cancer, but we hope this book assists you in achieving, and recognizing, personal peaks throughout the cancer struggle.

---

[2]Reprinted with permission of the National Rehabilitation Counseling Association.

Corrigan (2008) wrote regarding her own breast cancer that her e-mail had "to be upbeat so people won't worry too much and funny so they won't be scared to write back" (p. 93). Co-survivors know that we aren't the ones with cancer, so what do we do with our fear? What do we do with our trauma at the cancer diagnosis of a loved one? We have been given, or we take on, the work of trying to understand cancer as quickly as possible. In a play written to summarize research results (Mulcahy, Parry, & Glover, 2009), we hear from a father diagnosed with cancer:

> You're not prepared. When you get that diagnosis . . . the whole goes out of whack! Everything goes crazy! Your mind goes through the worst scenario. . . . It's just awful . . . we just deal with these horrible diagnoses and we don't have anything to help with something like that. (p. 32)

The researchers' conclusion: "Sometimes the person with cancer just needs someone to walk that road with them, even if neither of them knows exactly where they are going" (p. 40).

Whether survivor or co-survivor, the message of a new inspiring documentary, *The CaN'Tswer*—to move beyond fear—is a message we hope this book brings home to you: "Ten years after his leukemia diagnosis, Ryan is a survivor who is reluctant to take risks and move forward with his life. . . . A backpacking trip through the Andes Mountains changes him and his perception of his cancer experience from one of Survivor to Thriver" (http://www.pocketbunny.ca/tc/About_the_Film.html). To thrive doesn't have to mean becoming a mountain climber, but it does mean "to progress toward or realize a goal despite or because of circumstances" (http://www.merriam-webster.com/dictionary). In living beyond cancer, understanding the disease; finding support from family, friends, and treatment team members; and accepting the disease if it results in chronic illness or disability all contribute to recovery and thriving. Even if cancer results in the death of a loved one, learning from the cancer experience can contribute to your ability to thrive.

Relationships connect many of the authors of chapters in this book, as well as the authors and the editor—we have met through travels, through work, through a concern for family support in cancer. Several of the authors who share their personal experiences with cancer also relate how this experience has led to or informed their experience as professionals. The chapter authors are cancer survivors, co-survivors, and professionals in cancer intervention, health care, education, and psychology. These categories are not mutually exclusive. For instance, chapter author Alice F. Chang, Ph.D., is a cancer survivor, a clinical psychologist, and an author. In her excellent book *A Survivor's Guide to Breast Cancer*, she writes, "information is the single most important factor in diminishing psychological trauma for patients" (Chang & Spruill, 2000, p. 14). We believe this is also true for co-survivors.

The chapters in this book are written to bring information in a concise, easy-to-read and easy-to-use format. We share our personal and professional experiences through personal stories and experience-based case examples. We hope that our stories provide the understanding necessary for coping and guidance to shortcut your search for information and resources, thereby giving you knowledge (sooner, rather than later) that might prove helpful in coping with a loved one's cancer diagnosis and your own resulting trauma.

We direct you to selected resources that we have found useful (we have been told by cancer survivors and co-survivors that one problem they face is too much information!). As a co-survivor, I first had trouble deciding where to turn for information—was there a difference (or just duplication?) between information offered by the National Cancer Institute versus the American Cancer Society? Most importantly, as you read this book, we want you to know that you are not alone. While we may depend on science to cure cancer, relationships see us through treatment and beyond.

The Chapters. From bumping his head against the steering wheel in response to his diagnosis, to researching his disease, examining his options, and choosing his own treatment approach, chapter 1 author Mark Clark takes us on his cancer journey. Drawing on his strengths, among them a desire to learn, Mark tells us, "I began transcendence over the disease and was able to take my family with me," making the decision to "embrace life."

Sarah Sample, a social worker in a cancer center, outlines in chapter 2 the clinical course of cancer, integrating case studies that illustrate family concerns in different developmental stages of a family life cycle. She integrates her experience as a family caregiver with knowledge gained from her clinical practice, offering families both a map of the cancer journey and the opportunity to make new meanings through their experience.

In chapter 3, school psychologist Lena Gaddis describes how cancer can become a disability for young cancer survivors, particularly if cancer or side effects of cancer treatment affects their educational performance. Lena details the legal rights of children within the school setting, and provides resources for obtaining more information regarding the education of children who are cancer survivors.

I traveled to Finland in 2008 in order to learn more about how practitioners there work with families and cancer. Chapter 4 authors Mika Niemelä and Leena Väisänen share their experience of helping children understand parental cancer by providing family intervention. Mika and Leena explain the concerns children have and demonstrate, through a case example, how they address the "need to know" that children have when a parent is living with cancer—enabling young co-survivors to thrive.

Deirdre Cobb-Roberts demonstrates in chapter 5 the multiple roles many of us play as she interweaves personal narrative with research-based information on African American families and health care. We learn from her honesty and openness regarding the challenges of being a caregiver and a co-survivor of cancer. Her personal story demonstrates the role of faith in African American communities in coping with cancer and chronic illness (see also chapter 6). We rethink what cancer can mean when Deirdre tells us, "Mom and I have been given the opportunity to rediscover our relationship, a potentially lost opportunity if not for her illness."

In chapter 6, Monica Robinson shares "the beautiful part" of seeing her African American family "make things happen" in supporting her grandmother through cancer treatment. Monica's advice is to "jump on board, dig in, and do," but she also reminds us that families and co-survivors need to keep communicating—among themselves and with the cancer team. We feel Monica's joy and confidence when she declares, "our prayers are going up; blessings are coming down."

In chapter 7, Sharon Johnson draws on her experience as an American Indian, as a breast cancer survivor, as the mother of a cancer survivor, as a consultant experienced in cancer-related research, and as a rehabilitation counselor. She shares her pragmatic approach to dealing with cancer by addressing those diagnosed, and welcomes family to join in learning about and understanding the cancer journey.

Chapter 8 author Alice Chang, with Paul Donnelly, uses case examples, interwoven with a drama based on her own cancer story, to demonstrate cultural aspects of the cancer experience among Asian American families. We learn, for instance, the importance of understanding what may be acknowledged publicly and what may only be acknowledged privately, the need for culturally and linguistically appropriate support groups, and to respect the culturally different ways families cope with cancer. Alice's take-home message for coping with a chronic illness such as cancer: "Do the best you can each day; remember that some days are better than others!"

Alma Flores, Dina Martinez Tyson, Gloria San Miguel, and Claudia Aguado Loi work together through LUNA, Inc., a nonprofit organization serving Latino cancer survivors and their loved ones. LUNA's goals include enhancing the knowledge, coping skills, and ability to embrace hope for Spanish-speaking individuals touched by cancer. In chapter 9, co-authors Alma, Dina, Gloria, and Claudia share their collective experiences with individuals, support groups, and a capstone cancer experience for many—Camp Alegria. As one participant commented, "friendships I made at the camp have become part of my family and my desire to keep living."

Through both her personal experience and her work as a social worker, chapter 10 author Sarah Sample discusses issues facing Lesbian/Gay/

Bisexual/Transgendered (LGBT) families dealing with cancer—from fears of coming out, to connection and reduced sense of isolation when supported by those accepting of different sexual orientations. Case examples help us to understand the importance of understanding, support, community, and "family of choice."

Cancer allows for new connections to be made. In chapter 11, Ilkka Saarnio shares how the Internet brought him both information and new relationships, including one with co-author Lorraine Johnston, when first dealing with cancer. I chatted with Ilkka over tea in Helsinki, Finland, and, in listening to his story, felt how powerful our opportunities to know one another on a global scale can be. Professionals caution us to make sure we can trust information obtained via the Internet—this is important advice—but I find it heartwarming and exciting that an engineer reminds us through his cancer experience that we can also use technology to make personal connections.

Chapter 12 author Maria Figueroa shares her wisdom and experience in assisting families in securing financial assistance to pay for cancer treatment, and even transportation in order to receive treatment. Maria also reminds us that cancer can impact work—work affects insurance—insurance affects access to treatment. Her pragmatic approach to finding financial resources helps us all, survivors or co-survivors.

Rose Gordon exemplifies in chapter 13 new friends born via this book. Having read one of her earlier works, I contacted Rose via e-mail and invited her to write a chapter. Through e-mail, we realized that we shared common stories. November 2009 found us sharing stories not via e-mail but over breakfast in Pigeon Forge, Tennessee. In "Finding Strength and Celebrating Life," Rose writes a "love story" about friendship—about being friend enough to accept a loved one's decision to forego further cancer treatment.

The professional counselor can serve families by using counseling skills to address feelings, concerns, and coping skills, as well as find "unused opportunities" via the cancer journey. In chapter 14, Joyce DeVoss encourages families impacted by cancer to be proactive in addressing the needs of all family members and to consider including a professional counselor on the family care team.

In reflecting on her mother's life and battle with cancer, chapter 15 author Rebecca Paradies provides an important message often heard in the world of cancer: Live in the moment. She writes, "Cancer has given me a right to live more fully, to follow my passion, to experience this life the best way I can, and to honor my mother by attempting to live a more compassionate life." Rebecca's story also demonstrates how her career in helping others has been informed by her co-survivor cancer experience (see also chapters 2, 9, and 10).

Social worker Anne Mallett shares in chapter 16 her personal story of chronic illness, which includes surviving cancer. Anne's story illustrates the importance of obtaining second opinions, self-determination, self-confidence, and the support of family and friends, giving us all courage to move forward in our search for health care—and in life—as our body, mind, and spirit tell us.

I am very grateful to the authors of the chapters in this book. It is their words that you will read and their experiences, both personal and professional, that comprise the content of this work. I am grateful to my husband, Ric Steffel, for his patience and sustenance while my dream of editing this book required me to ignore him. I thank Deborah Carvalko at Praeger for her immediate interest in and support of this work when I first proposed it. I also want to thank friend and colleague Professor Elizabeth Kendall, co-editor of *Disability Insights and Issues*, for her insightful comments and review of chapters, as well as for writing the Foreword for this first book of our new series. Finally, I would like to acknowledge the skill and amicable spirit of Denise Stanley, project manager, Cadmus Communications, in watching over the production of this book, to include the fine work of Jodie Littleton, copyeditor.

References

A National Action Plan for Cancer Survivorship: Advancing Public Health Strategies. (2004). The Centers for Disease Control and Prevention, National Center for Chronic Disease Prevention and Health Promotion, Division of Cancer Prevention and Control and the Lance Armstrong Foundation.

Chan, F., da Silva Cardoso, E., Copeland, J., Jones, R., & Fraser, R. T. (2009). Workplace accommodations. In M. Feuerstein (Ed.), *Work and cancer survivors* (pp. 233–254). New York: Springer.

Chan, F., Strauser, D., da Silva Cardoso, E., Xi Zheng, L., Chan, J. Y. C., & Feuerstein, M. (2008). State vocational services and employment in cancer survivors. *Journal of Cancer Survivorship, 2,* 169–178.

Chang, A. F., & Spruill, K. M. (2000). *A survivor's guide to breast cancer: A chronic illness specialist tells you what to expect and shares the inspiring account of her own experiences as a patient.* Oakland: New Harbinger Publications.

Corrigan, K. (2008). *The middle place.* New York: Voice, Hyperion.

Gilgun, J. F. (1992). Definitions, methodologies, and methods in qualitative family research. In J. F. Gilgun, K. Daly, & G. Handel (Eds.) *Qualitative methods in family research* (pp. 22–39). Newbury Park, CA: Sage.

Hanson, K., & Kriescher, M. (2006). *Cancer survivorship: State policy issues.* Washington, DC: National Conference of State Legislatures, The Forum for America's Ideas [www.ncsl.org].

Hewitt, M., Greenfield, S., & Stovall, E. (Eds.) (2005). *From cancer patient to cancer survivor: Lost in transition.* Report from the Committee on Cancer Survivorship: Improving Care and Quality of Life, Institute of Medicine and National Research Council. Washington, DC: National Academies Press.

Johnson, S. (2009). *Peaks and valleys: Making good and bad times work for you—at work and in life.* New York: Atria Books.

Marshall, C. A. (2008). Family and culture: Using autoethnography to inform rehabilitation practice with cancer survivors. *Journal of Applied Rehabilitation Counseling, 39*(1), 9–19.

Mulcahy, C. M., Parry, D. C., & Glover, T. D. (2009). Between diagnosis and death: A performance text about cancer, shadows, and the ghosts we cannot escape. *International Review of Qualitative Research, 2*(1), 29–42.

Power, P. W. (1995). Family. In A. E. Dell Orto & R. P. Marienelli, *Encyclopedia of disability and rehabilitation.* New York: Simon & Schuster.

Pransky, G. (2009). Foreword. In M. Feuerstein, *Work and cancer survivors* (pp. vii–viii). New York: Springer.

Stager, P. (2009). We can cry later: A story of surviving cancer. In C. A. Marshall, E. Kendall, M. E. Banks, & R. M. S. Gover (Eds.), *Disabilities: Insights from across fields and around the world: Vol 1. The experience: Definitions, causes, and consequences* (pp. 81–85). Westport, CT: Praeger.

Sutherland, G., Dpsych, L. H., White, V. Jefford, M., & Hegarty, S. (2008). How does a cancer education program impact on people with cancer and their family and friends? *Journal of Cancer Education, 23*(2), 126–132.

Verbeek, J., & Spelten, E. (2007). Work. In M. Feuerstein (Ed.), *Handbook of cancer survivorship* (pp. 381–396). New York: Springer.

CHAPTER 1

My Journey: Learning What Matters

Mark Clark

wo thousand seven was a horrible year, yet it was a year that made me closer to my family. I now have a greater understanding of my place in my family. Like all cancer patients, I live with uncertainty, but this uncertainty has empowered my life, not diminished it. I now have different values and priorities. My universe has moved. My family thinks I am a better person.

In March 2007, I was diagnosed with colon cancer. Although I had harbored a strong suspicion that I had colon cancer, I was emotionally unprepared for the diagnosis. I was most notably underprepared for the response of my treating general practitioner, who was even less prepared for the diagnosis than I was. He had expected that the results of my tests would reveal his patient to be an overanxious middle-aged male who was extremely stressed, but not physically ill. No doubt, he thought that his patient was more in need of antidepressants than surgery. But here we were, at the beginning of a journey through shadows occasioned by the odd bright shining light. One of us, at least, was going to be changed dramatically by this event.

After the emotional discovery of the diagnosis and frenzied telephone calls to a surgeon's receptionist, I left the doctor's office for my car. I had driven to the doctor's office alone. I had felt assured that I would be able to handle this matter and, even though I had very high suspicions that

I was in "tiger country," I did not think the tiger was actually going to be on top of me. This was "game on." I felt cut in halves. One half was going through the mechanistic movements that one must do to move from one place to another; the other half had exited the world for an unknown place between the living and the dead.

My car—my pride and joy—was now a mere object, my universe inverted. I felt betrayed by my biology and isolated from the normalcy that I now envy in people. I sat in my car and bumped my forehead against the steering wheel. I was not in control of anything. I had been emotionally stripped and placed somewhere in isolation from the rest of the living world of hope.

My trip home was a blur. Should I have been driving? Definitely not! I managed the drive, but I did not go straight home. I telephoned my sister, who was with my mother, and told her of the diagnosis. My sister's reaction was like a cannon shell exploding around me—an emotional outpouring of grief that I had only seen in the bereaved. My 80-year-old mother would have to be told; I did not have the strength to do so. I delegated that to my sister.

Next was to contact my wife. It was as if I were working from the outer perimeter to the inner sanctum of my life. My sons needed to be told. I arrived home and managed to tell my wife, my world imploding. After that, I moved on to my sons. One, a nurse, seemed to take it better than the other, a lawyer.

My fear escalated and penetrated to the bone. My head spun more than the wheel on a Formula One racing car. My thoughts were interspersed with disbelief and complete shock. How could this be? I had plans, my career, expectations. . . . Cancer happened to others, but surely not me. Yet I was in God's waiting room, never having known I was in the neighborhood.

Time went on. The visit to the surgeon was reassuring, but I was still fearful. A phony peace broke out, but I was still penetrated by moments of panic. There was little likelihood of my needing chemotherapy, as the cancer in my bowel was small. It did not appear to have penetrated the bowel wall. Everything was upbeat, but surreal. I began to dread the surgery, not the cancer.

I was preoccupied, selfishly, with myself. I started to notice a difference in my immediate circle. I was drifting from the world of relevance to irrelevance in some quarters. People from work had lunch with me—everybody was very jovial and convivial. Only after I left the lunch did I understand—it was a living wake! I had sung my song in their eyes, and I was now being kindly supported offstage. It was as if they were saying good-bye. There was no expectation that I would be back at work. I was only on sick leave, but clearly others thought it was likely to be a more permanent absence.

My family began to circle the wagons or, perhaps more accurately, gather around me as elephants do when one of the herd is in distress.

My inner circle was drawing close while some on the periphery were pulling away. My faith in fellow human beings was now mixed. Some people were moving away, while others, hitherto unknown to me, were moving close, committing great acts of kindness.

I was not well placed to understand the anguish of my family; they did not disclose their feelings to me. I realized that I needed to prepare my will and tidy up other things one would do if going away on a long holiday. I was largely self-absorbed.

The surgery went well. The surgeon was upbeat for about a week, but then the lab results came back. My very red-eyed surgeon told me that the cancer had managed to penetrate a single lymph node. The risk that it had gotten away was there. It was aggressive as well. My odds for survival took a tumble, but they were still with me. I felt as if I had been dropped from the ninth floor of a building. My eldest son, the nurse, was with me when I received the news. He was very distressed. Chemotherapy was necessary. I began a fight for my life.

During my recovery from surgery, I drew on my strengths—for instance, my desire to learn. As a child, I had had a poor education and did not complete high school. I was treated rather cruelly by the school system and left at the first opportunity. However, as a detective on the police force, I attended the university part time and began the grind toward a degree.

I researched the disease. While the information that I found was not very reassuring, I examined the options. I chose an aggressive approach using an experimental drug, as well as the usual treatment. I began an attack on the cancer based upon the best rational decisions that I could make. I began transcendence over the disease and was able to take my family with me. I looked for scientific support that I could include in my treatment regime and located a former research scientist who helped me with diet and nutritional issues. He also educated me about my immune system. I telephoned and spoke to the team from the company that supplied the experimental drug. I checked the dosages with them.

I also checked the stock market reports on the experimental drug. The market reaction when the company reported on this drug was very positive, with a rise in the stock price. I assumed that "hard-headed" capitalists were not likely to invest money in a losing product. In any case, the market would scrutinize any new drug so thoroughly that a poor performer would be identified very quickly. The market had access to real-time information and would react accordingly to correct the price. So I let the market do research for me. I drew on all available systems of information to produce an intelligence-driven treatment program for myself. In doing this, I began to reverse the very thing that was undermining me and my family—the loss of personal power and relevance.

This loss following a cancer diagnosis can be the most powerful punch of the disease. Disempowerment radiates from the individual to the entire family. The individual can retreat into a cocoon in order to isolate the self from the reality of mortality. We are not the people we once were. Our vitality is lost in a sea of despair. Our disconnection from the world is reflected in our relationships. We no longer engage in conversations with people about their lives. We are awash in our own self-interest or, dare I say, in my case, self-pity. When we transcend this cocoon—this loss of power—we enable our family to do so as well.

I drew upon my early drill instructors, who would not let me feel sorry for myself. I would hear them in my mind. Meaningful relationships are not possible in the face of disempowerment. I had to move past disempowerment—to engage and challenge—if I were to support my family and reconnect with them in a positive way. My health, or rather my reaction to my health, was shutting down their joy of life. Cancer was winning on all fronts. My decision: I might not survive cancer, but I could embrace life. I then began to reconnect to the workplace. Suddenly, I had visitors from work. The topic moved from cancer to what was happening at work. I was back in the game.

My regime was rigid. Although I was very weak, I made sure that I exercised during chemo. I did not want my muscles to waste. I exercised when I felt like curling up in a ball and crying. I stuck to my diet, although my mouth tasted like some metallic substance had been poured into it. My body reinvented itself. My spirit grew stronger. The stronger it grew, the greater lift my family felt. I am living the wisdom that no man is an island.

When ill, my contribution—the contribution my life had made—was very important to me. Cancer made this very relevant for me. I had not pondered my legacy as profoundly before. I had always wanted to do worthy work, but cancer had me counting the chips on the table. As a cancer survivor, the words of Kenny Rogers in "The Gambler" resonated within me: "You never count your money when you're sittin' at the table. There'll be time enough for countin' when the dealing's done." It is not yet time for me to count my chips; I am still playing the game, but with a different focus. Like most people, I am not without self-interest, but a major question for me now is, "What can I do for others?" I owe for my survival thus far.

CHAPTER 2

Making New Meanings: Cancer and the Family

Sarah Sample

I picked up the phone. My brother said, "It's Mom. She had to have surgery this morning. She's got cancer. You need to come." That was 21 years ago. I was 34 years old. Everything changed for me from that moment. Several years later, my phone rang. My father said, "It's your sister-in-law. She has cancer. We better go—that's what our family does." I knew we had to go and that for my 11- and 9-year-old nieces, life would change from that moment.

Advances in treatments for some cancers have resulted in an overall reduction in cancer mortality. Cancer, while still feared as a life-threatening illness, in many cases is now seen as a chronic illness rather than as a terminal disease. As a result, quality of life and survivorship have become a focus of research and intervention in recent years. Given that the family plays an important role in the patient's quality of life, it is important to understand the impact of cancer on family. Family life is significantly different after cancer than before. There is now a deeper understanding of how a cancer diagnosis impacts family and friends throughout the cancer journey. Cancer affects us in diverse ways, colored in part by our age, our unique relationship to loved ones, our stage of life development, and the supports we have available to us.

It is estimated that three out of four families will be impacted to some degree by cancer (Veach, Nicholas, & Barton, 2002). Yet families often enter this unfamiliar territory without a clear map of the journey. Based on my experiences as a daughter, sister-in-law, and friend of those diagnosed with cancer, as well as my work as an oncology social worker for more than 20 years, I hope in this chapter to provide families who are embarking on the cancer journey with knowledge, understanding, and new meanings about the impact of cancer on their lives.

As for me, I had believed that my mother would live forever. After her diagnosis, and with the new knowledge and understanding that life was fragile, I began to look at my intimate relationships in new ways. For instance, my relationship with my father was significantly affected. Indeed, after I received the call that my mother had cancer, the life that I had planned was changed, and I was propelled into a career of helping others facing cancer.

Understanding Families and Cancer

When I counsel patients and families facing cancer, it helps me to know who belongs in the family, where the family is in its developmental stage, and the stage they have reached in the cancer journey. Are they a young couple in the beginning of building a life together, with new careers disrupted by lengthy and intensive treatment? Are they a young family dealing with a dying parent? Are they a recently retired couple that planned to travel and relax in their later years and now are faced with a diagnosis of advanced cancer? Juxtaposing the clinical course of cancer with family developmental stage provides a framework to understand what the impact of cancer might be, how the family may cope, and how I may be of service to both the patient and the family.

Here I begin by defining the family as a system. Next I explain the stages of a family life cycle and then, through describing the clinical course of cancer, illustrate some of the ways that cancer can impact the family. The clinical course of cancer, which may include initial diagnosis, treatment, rehabilitation, survivorship (remission or cure), recurrence, and end of life, will have different impacts depending on where the family is in its life cycle, family support, geographic location, and historical patterns of coping in the family. The degree of impact is affected by many factors, including the timing of diagnosis in the family life cycle, the seriousness of the diagnosis, the openness of the family unit, and the individual position in the family of the person diagnosed. For instance, the experience for a child who has a parent with cancer (see chapter 4) will be markedly different from that of an adult who has a parent with cancer.

Family Systems: Definition and Principles

A family is regarded as a system. Families are diverse and might include members who are biologically related, or not; have opposite or same-sex partnerships; and exist with or without children (Lewis, 2006). A family might be described as single parent; nuclear and heterosexual; lesbian, gay, bisexual, and transgendered (LGBT; see chapter 10); multigenerational; couples; and so on. Irrespective of their makeup, families are composed of people who have a shared history, a shared lineage, and a shared future. Families are also emotional systems (Kerr, 1981).

Individuals and relationships are shaped by family. Family stories shape our understanding of what illness is about. A history of cancer in the family will inform the family's responses to the cancer diagnosis and treatment. Family cancer stories might be influenced by socioeconomic status, culture, ethnicity, gender differences, history of coping, and sexual orientation.

Family structure, the coping abilities of each individual member, and the coping of the family as a whole, affect how the family is impacted by cancer. Ironically, during the crisis of cancer when stress levels are at their highest, the family is called upon to function at its best. Because family members mutually influence each other, when one individual in the family system is affected by cancer, it more often than not causes disturbances/change in the rest of the family system, as well as between the family system and the health care system (Rolland, 2005).

Cancer can impact the family in three major ways: change future plans, upset the usual patterns of communication within the family, and alter external connections with the world (Cassileth & Hamilton, 1979). Change can be seen in that parents may be less available to their children, roles may be changed (a daughter may take her father to the doctor), and relationships may be affected. The family's standard of living may decrease due to economic burdens from either direct or hidden costs of cancer. Uncertainty, a sense of helplessness, and loss of control are often experienced, creating instability in how the family usually operates as members attempt to adapt to changed lives. Roles and functions are also strengthened and supported by societal and gender norms often set by the specific community or culture.

Case Example: A Daughter's Role—Present and Supportive

My mother's diagnosis of cancer was a shock to our whole family and was the first cancer experience for all of us. As the only daughter, and assumed to be single (see chapter 10), I was expected to fly across the country, leaving my university studies to become my parents' primary caregiver. This role was expected of me based on the history, structure, and function of our family over generations. My brothers had the choice to respond as they chose, whereas I was expected to be present and supportive. My brothers continued with their work—they were not able or willing to function as caregivers. On several occasions I "overfunctioned," taking on too much responsibility. For instance, my father, who experienced his second heart failure during this time, was admitted to the same hospital where my mother was being treated for cancer. One day I found myself going back and forth for most of the day between the emergency room and my mother's hospital room because both parents were worried about how the other was doing—I was the communicator. On that day I realized what was happening and asked one of my brothers to come to the hospital to assist me.

Family history and beliefs, as well as the meanings attached to those beliefs, influence how the family responds to a cancer diagnosis. Beliefs and the way a family manages illness may be passed through many generations. Family beliefs and their emotional intensity can be very powerful because the family is an emotional system. For example, some families believe that illness is an emotional or mental weakness. A belief such as this may impede the family members' ability to adequately support one another.

If cancer led to death in a family over generations, the family belief is likely that cancer always leads to death. Early in my clinical work, I remember counseling a woman whose mother had been hospitalized with a bowel obstruction. I realized halfway through our session that I was basing my counseling direction on the belief that her mother would die. I became aware that my belief was just that: my belief, and not necessarily my client's belief. I became aware that just because my mother died of cancer does not mean all mothers die of cancer.

In my work I have met family members who believe, more than the patient themselves, that if their family member is optimistic and positive the cancer may be cured, while if their family member is negative and pessimistic the cancer will return. This belief can place a huge burden on the patient. A predominant belief of many families is that stress causes cancer; therefore, stress must be eradicated from family life. Unresolved issues of blame, shame, or guilt can strongly affect views of the cause or cure of cancer and how the family adapts.

Remembering, then, that families are complex systems, a brief overview of stages in a family life cycle follows. The family life cycle example is based on a North American/Western model, yet it provides a beginning framework from which to look at the clinical course of cancer and its subsequent impact on the family. Different cultures, of course, may have different ways of experiencing family life (see chapters 5–9).

Understanding Implications of the Family Life Cycle and Cancer

There are specific tasks to complete in each developmental stage of the family life cycle (Veach et al., 2002). Normally, times of transition from one phase to the next in the family life cycle are periods of upheaval and confusion. There are adjustments to new responsibilities, new roles, and new boundaries. If cancer arrives during these transition times, there may be even more upheaval and even greater adjustments to be made. Thus it is important to remember that when a family member is diagnosed with cancer, it has not only a unique impact on each individual, but also on family relationships within a given stage of the life cycle.

Gender-role socialization has been integrated with the family life cycles stages to provide a more in-depth understanding about relationships involving female cancer patients and their families (Petersen, Kruczek, & Shaffner, 2003).

Cancer can disrupt the development of the family life cycle and increase instability of each stage. It often leads to confusion and creates separation or entanglement in families. Each individual within the family may be dealing with her or his own emotions and anxiety and feel unprepared to meet the needs of the person with cancer. However, a crisis of cancer can also lead to healing within a family; family members discover strength and resilience they never knew they had—they find new ways of being together and find new meanings in life.

Single Young Adult

Discussion of the family life cycle now includes the development of single individuals because the percentage of single-person households has risen dramatically since the 1990s (McGoldrick & Carter, 1999). During this stage, the young adult is learning to balance connectedness and separateness with his or her family of origin. Young adults are learning to identify with their family of origin while also developing a stronger sense of self in connection with others outside the family. They may move out to live on their own or remain in the parent's home. Young adults are beginning careers, exploring the world, or continuing with education. A cancer diagnosis can halt the development of peer relationships and career goals.

New Couple

A couple starts to date. In time, the couple begins to form a new system separate from their families of origin, and each grows more accepting of his or her emotional and financial responsibility. As well as committing to each other, there is a process of joining two or more families of origin. Values, beliefs, and issues surrounding religion, intimacy, money, relationships, illness, and work are part of this process of joining. When one member of the couple is diagnosed with cancer, stress on the newly formed partnership may bring instability and the potential for breakdown of the relationship. Returning home to be cared for by parents after one has been independent can halt the process of this stage of family development. The couple then may not have the space, independence, or alone time to grow as a couple. The relationship can break down or it can be strengthened.

Families with Young Children

This is a time when parents are intensely involved in childrearing duties. The family's task is to accept new members while juggling individual needs, the marriage, the extended family, and the outside world. Depending on the family's makeup, the impact of cancer may be more or less significant. The ill parent can lose a sense of feeling needed. Potential disruptions may include the well parent being overwhelmed by added responsibilities, difficulties in carrying out childrearing tasks, meeting financial responsibilities, and meeting challenges of work and other relationships. Role changes in childrearing tasks and adjustment to new responsibilities for the whole family will need to be negotiated. If the patient had been the main source of family income, or if a couple has relied on two incomes and now has only one, financial stress is increased. These adjustments cause strain emotionally and functionally on the system as a whole. Children may show behavior changes because they are worried about the sick parent, worried that they caused their parent's illness, that they may be left alone, or that they might get cancer too (see chapter 4).

Families with Adolescents

This developmental stage is often a time of major reorganization, confusion, and intensity for the family. Adolescents need to begin to move toward increased independence to gain a sense of self and autonomy, and begin to separate from their parents. Adolescents are undergoing physical, emotional, and sexual changes. With a cancer diagnosis, increased demands placed on adolescents may result in stalling their individual development. They may need to take care of younger siblings. They may react by becoming too involved in the family illness—overfunctioning—or by prematurely withdrawing from the family. They might display serious behavior problems or have difficulties in school. The family may need to adjust to extended family or friends coming into the home to help care for the ill parent.

Families Launching Children

Another significant family time of change is when children begin to leave home. When all the children are gone, the empty nest returns the focus to the parent or marital couple. This is often the longest phase of the family life cycle. It is another time of changing roles and redefining relationships. Children are away building their own careers and/or families, but they may be drawn back by the cancer experience to parents who may depend on them more, especially if they are elderly and/or have a disability. When cancer comes into the family, adult children may be faced with the challenge of moving forward in their own lives while also needing to care for a parent who is ill. If families live at a distance from each other, they may experience more anxiety and helplessness because they aren't able to give direct care and support to their loved one.

Families Later in Life

Depending on socioeconomic status, retirement for couples later in life can begin a time of relaxation and travel—enjoying a slower, simpler life together. Retirement can also be a time when a couple struggles financially with fixed or limited income resources. Older adults are more likely to begin to accept their own mortality; it is a time when one can expect to face the death of a partner as well. There is an increased risk of cancer and other chronic diseases. While relationships with grandchildren and great-grandchildren may be a focus of joy for families later in life, adult children may also need to care for elderly parents.

Understanding the Clinical Course of Cancer

Because there are as many stories as there are families, it is impossible to offer a specific map of the ways in which cancer impacts families. Exploring the phases of the clinical course of cancer in conjunction with the developmental stage of the family can be useful in understanding fully how cancer can impact families. The clinical course of cancer affects the severity of the demands on family. In early stage cancers, the impact will be minimal depending on the history of the cancer experience in the family. Aggressive cancers, later stage cancers, or recurrence of cancer will impose more demands and greater disruptions.

Fluctuations throughout the clinical course are often described as a roller coaster ride (Holland & Lewis, 2001). I hear patients and families use this metaphor—the roller coaster—when struggling to find ways to stay on the ride with all its ups and downs. I hear family caregivers include themselves as part of the treatment and say that "we" are receiving chemotherapy or radiation therapy, reinforcing our understanding that cancer is an ordeal experienced by the family and not the patient alone.

Four different clinical paths follow a suspicion of cancer (Holland & Lewis, 2001). The first path is diagnosis, primary treatment (surgery, chemotherapy, radiation, or hormonal therapies), rehabilitation, long-term survival, and cure. On the second path, the patient may undergo treatment and enjoy a time of remission, but then experience a recurrence of cancer and another course of treatment. On the third path, the treatment for recurrence fails and palliative measures are taken to relieve symptoms. The fourth clinical path, one for which no curative effort is possible, can be identified upon diagnosis, during treatment, or when recurrence occurs. On this fourth clinical path, treatment is aimed at controlling symptoms and maximizing quality of life; once it is determined that no curative effort is possible, the time to death can be very short or can be quite lengthy. Here, I focus on the clinical course of the first path.

Diagnostic Phase

After hearing, comprehending, and understanding the diagnosis, the next task is to make treatment decisions (see chapter 1). Patients and families are in shock. They enter into a world of unpredictability and may experience a sense of loss of control and helplessness. Family members, no matter the prognosis, may begin to experience anticipatory grief.

Existential questions can surface. The diagnosis of cancer brings up end-of-life concerns and worries for most people, regardless of the prognosis or the stage of cancer at diagnosis. Similar to that of some patients, family members, upon hearing of a cancer diagnosis, are also gripped by fear of the possibility of their loved one's death. For a new couple starting a life together and with plans for a future, a cancer diagnosis can put a tremendous amount of strain on the relationship. It can either strengthen or weaken the relationship.

Case Example: Tom and Kathi's Story. Tom and his girlfriend, Kathi, came to see me when he was first diagnosed, early in their relationship. Both were in shock. They were told that Tom would need surgery, radiation, and chemotherapy to treat a rare type of sarcoma and would likely have a limp for the rest of his life. Kathi said that all she could think of was that Tom could die. Kathi appeared significantly more distressed than Tom and said she didn't know what to do or how to help—she felt angry because of the unpredictability of the situation. On the other hand, Tom stated that his biggest distress was that he was going to have a limp for the rest of his life—not that he could die. Tom hopes to search for understanding the meaning of this crisis. The couple met each other's respective parents for the first time during his treatment. Neither of them expected to meet their families this way. Kathi struggles to work full time and take care of Tom. She feels overwhelmed and exhausted, and continues to worry about both Tom and their future.

I have found very often in my clinical practice that the partner is much more distressed than the patient. While the focus for the patient is on treatment and doing something about the cancer, the family member feels that he or she has no control and thus focuses more on fear of the unknown. Although Tom and Kathi were devastated by the cancer diagnosis, through counseling sessions, they now express how they have come to know each other on a deeper level, have realized that they work well together as a new couple in the face of a life crisis, and acknowledge that they have greater appreciation and love for each other.

Treatment Phase: Treatment or No Treatment Possible

The primary treatment for cancer can include surgery, chemotherapy, radiation, and hormonal or immunotherapy. It can also include watching and waiting. Depending on the type and stage of cancer, treatment can be as short as one surgery or can last months and years. If treatment is lengthy, the patient endures tests, scans, and biopsies while the family struggles to remain on the roller coaster ride. Day-to-day life with cancer can be a long haul. If someone in the family needs to attend daily radiation treatments, each day will need to be organized around treatment time. The side effects of chemotherapy and radiation often accumulate, and the family will likely need to increase both practical and emotional support to get through treatment. The treatment course can have an impact on the patient's physical abilities and energy levels, with increasing workload on family. This can put stress on the family as a whole. Family members often want to protect each other from difficult emotions and the fear of death while enduring treatment. The family may struggle with differing approaches to health care decisions, coping styles, and financial and work-related concerns. There is also the possibility that no treatment is recommended. In cases of slow growing cancers, such as a low-grade non-Hodgkin's lymphoma, patients are in the watch-and-wait mode for months, and sometimes years. This uncertainty in the future may cause ongoing anxiety for the family.

Case Example: Andrea's Story. Andrea is a 24-year-old student and the primary caregiver for her mother, Barbara, who is undergoing breast cancer treatment. Barbara also has a history of depression and has attempted suicide twice in the past; she entered an alcohol treatment center a number of years ago and remains sober. Barbara separated from her husband when Andrea was 10 years old. Andrea is the youngest child and has three older brothers. Andrea lives with her partner of one year just a short distance from her mother; she spends most days taking care of Barbara. Barbara experiences significant anxiety, worry, and ambivalence about her chemotherapy treatment and believes that painful cancer experiences she has witnessed in close relatives and friends contribute to her fear of her own treatment process. Barbara is currently on a number of medications for depression and anxiety.

Andrea came to see me because she is overwhelmed with the burden of taking care of her mother. Andrea states that her mother expects her to care for her both emotionally and functionally on a daily basis. At the same time, Barbara is verbally abusive toward Andrea. Developmentally, Andrea became the overfunctioning, responsible person in the family, and she now feels guilty if she is away from her mother. With Barbara's cancer, an old pattern of family roles and responsibilities has resurfaced, and Andrea feels she cannot abandon her mother. Yet she feels resentful that her brothers are not doing their share. Caregiving has become a full-time job for Andrea while she is on a summer break from college. The daily care of her mother is now impacting Andrea's relationship with her partner. It is also detrimental to her career goals, as she feels summer jobs related to her field of work are necessary for keeping up with her classmates. She worries that this may impact her ability to find work when she finishes school.

Through counseling sessions, Andrea was able to gain insight and understanding about how she functions in her relationship with her mother. She realized that old beliefs and patterns were resurfacing during the cancer journey. By releasing these old beliefs, Andrea began to feel less guilty. Even though her mother continues to expect more from her, Andrea has found different ways to support her mother while still continuing to pursue her career and build her relationship with her partner. Andrea has found a new sense of strength and growth within herself as an individual separate from her mother.

Rehabilitation, Recovery, Remission

Following treatment, there is a time to recover physically, mentally, and emotionally. Often it comes as a surprise that the emotional and mental roller coaster ride continues after treatment. Families may wonder if life will ever be the same again. Fears of recurrence can trouble the family. What if they didn't get it all? Any aches or pains experienced cause the patient and family members to panic. With time, the patient gradually begins to return to responsibilities, adapting to any ongoing side effects of treatment and returning to work. There is a gradual resumption of family roles and function—often a major adjustment for the family.

It is hard to be immersed in the cancer experience and then suddenly return to a world that exists outside of the illness. Families struggle to regain some sense of normalcy. This time after treatment is often described by patient and family as "living in limbo." The family wants life to be as it once was, but life is not the same as before cancer. The process of physical, mental, and emotional recovery can extend well beyond the last treatment. Recovery after treatment can be a difficult time for a young family.

Case Example: Jessica and Liz's Story. Jessica is a 37-year-old lesbian woman who recently finished treatment for breast cancer. Jessica and her partner, Liz, have a 5-year-old daughter, Sara. It was hard for Jessica to hear her diagnosis of an agresssive breast cancer; during and after treatment, her biggest fear was dying—not seeing her daughter grow up. Because Jessica is a physician herself, she says she knows too much. Her anxiety and fear of death overwhelm her. Although her oncologist told the couple that Jessica was being treated with curative intent, Jessica still fears the worst. Just prior to her diagnosis, the couple was planning for Jessica to bring a sister or brother into the world for Sara. The cancer diagnosis brought their plans for a growing family to a halt—a huge loss for the couple. During treatment, Liz was caring and supportive and took on more child care responsibilities. She expressed anger while Jessica expressed more worry and anxiety about the future. Now that treatment has ended, Liz is angry more than ever and wants "the whole situation" to go away.

This family is struggling to achieve a "new normal." Jessica is returning to an exercise routine, spending time with Sara—returning to her role and responsibilities as a parent. Liz is relieved of her double parental duty, but worries more than Jessica about the cancer returning. Jessica still has bouts of tears at times when she looks at her daughter and wonders about the future. She has discovered meditation—something she never thought she would do. Meditation has helped her live in the moment, find new ways of seeing, and appreciate her life. Liz and Jessica, living with the uncertainty of their future, try to maintain hope and continue with their lives and their devotion to Sara.

Long-term Survivorship

In long-term survivorship, the family often struggles to find a new normal with a deeper sense and understanding of mortality. It can be a time of increased appreciation for life and family. At the same time, there is a new awareness of cancer hanging over the family—what has been described as "living under the sword of Damocles" (Veach et al., 2002). Families may experience increasing anxiety and fears of an uncertain future. The question is often asked, "After treatment, what next?" Children may be challenged, particularly if the parents are experiencing grief, loss, and difficulty in their "new normal." Generally, families want things to remain the same. Families want familiarity. However, cancer disrupts the system, launching it into an unfamiliar landscape. Fears, anxiety, and worries can echo throughout the family.

Case Example: Theresa's Story. Theresa is a 63-year-old divorced woman who was diagnosed with colon cancer. Theresa has two daughters and two sons ranging in age from 19 to 27. She is of Filipino and Spanish decent and had been married to a Canadian. Her children were born in Canada and have adopted North American culture. Throughout her treatment, when Theresa experienced severe depression and anxiety, the entire family's anxiety intensified. She regularly let her children know that in her culture it is expected that family members play a major role in taking care of each other. Her four children lead busy lives, some with families of their own and careers, yet they still managed to schedule time for their mother on a regular basis. This was a devoted and loving family who described themselves as overly close, particularly during Theresa's cancer journey. After treatment, Theresa continued to experience severe bouts of depression. There were times of breakdown in communication within the family. Theresa's son Mark was most sensitive to his mother's inability to move on with her life. He had already interrupted his career and wanted to get on with his life, but he felt guilty about it. They had ongoing fights and communication difficulties. Mark frequently called on his brother and sisters to help. Although Theresa was doing well since treatment, she relied on her children more than ever. Theresa's fear of recurrence was hanging over the whole family.

Through individual and family counseling sessions, Theresa became more aware of her own strengths and has relied less on her children. Her children have become less worried about their mother and thus are able to devote more attention to their own lives. Mark found ways to support his mother and continue with his career. He even accepted a job outside the country. Theresa is enjoying her grandchildren and has found new meaning for her own life by finding ways to leave a legacy for her family—she is writing her life story.

Conclusion

It is acknowledged that cancer results in death for some, and that the end stage of life can be the most difficult and emotionally intense time for a family. However, as death and dying are not the focus of this book, a discussion of cancer as a terminal illness, the benefits of palliative care, and family bereavement are not included in this chapter. However, it is true that families deal with losses throughout the clinical course of cancer—losses such as past activities and abilities, and certain expectations for the future—even with cancer that does not result in death. Former experiences with loss in the family will play a part in the experience of any current loss. For many families, anticipating loss together, facing loss together, and helping each other get through the process can be very healing and powerful.

The family may cope better and experience less impact throughout the cancer experience if, for instance, individual difference is tolerated, parents maintain rules and boundaries, and children maintain age-appropriate responsibilities such as continuing with their education and after-school activities. The family that discusses cancer and its implications for family life together can feel strengthened to face all the challenges that cancer brings. Flexibility of roles and rules during changes and transitions throughout the family life cycle can lessen any negative impact. If distancing or cutting off relationships is not used to solve problems, the impact on family will be lessened.

The family facing cancer will test its ability to cope. The crisis of a cancer diagnosis and treatment can bring some family members new opportunities for more satisfying and fulfilling relationships. Some families find meaning in the cancer experience and develop an understanding of a greater purpose. Despite high levels of distress, families can have positive experiences. If the family has healthy, open communication, it can adjust well, and members are more likely to find deeper meaning and connection to themselves and others throughout the cancer journey.

One day my mother was having great difficulty descending the stairs in her house to reach her favorite chair. When she finally got there, I asked if she would like me to wash and massage her feet. As I sat at her feet, comforting her, I was overcome with a closeness and connection that I had never felt before with her. When she told me she felt as if she could run up and down the stairs a hundred times after I had finished, I was overwhelmed with tears. I didn't know such a simple act could be so powerful and meaningful to both of us.

When my mother was diagnosed with cancer and was receiving treatment in the hospital, most health professionals were not able see the pain and distress of family members. No one asked how I was doing or how the family was coping. Now, after working with families and cancer for more than 20 years, I have come to think of that experience as an offering to me that I accepted. I was propelled to work in oncology because of the experience of cancer in my family. I am grateful and deeply appreciative that the work I do with patients and families living with cancer allows me every day to discover and rediscover my true compassionate self. Thus families may find new meaning and strengths in coping with the cancer crisis and, as co-survivors, may find a heightened sense of being alive and a greater awareness of life's preciousness and purpose.

References

Cassileth, B. R., & Hamilton, J. (1979). The family with cancer. In B. Cassileth (Ed.), *The cancer patient: Social and medical aspects of care* (pp. 233–247). Philadelphia: Lea & Febiger.

Holland, J., & Lewis, S. (2001). *The human side of cancer: Living with hope, coping with uncertainty*. New York: Harper Collins.

Kerr, M. (1981). Cancer and the family emotional system. In J. Goldberg (Ed.), *Psychotherapeutic treatment of the cancer patient* (pp. 273–314). New York: Free Press.

Lewis, F. M. (2006). The effects of cancer survivorship on families and caregivers: More research is needed on long-term survivors. *Cancer Nursing, 29* (Suppl. 2), 20–25.

McGoldrick, M., & Carter, B. (1999). *The expanded family life cycle: Individual, family and social perspectives*. Boston: Allyn & Bacon.

Petersen, L., Kruczek, T., & Shaffner, A. (2003.) Gender roles and the family life cycle: The case of women with cancer. In A. Lyuness & M. Prouty (Eds.), *Feminist perspectives in medical family therapy* (pp. 99–119). New York: Haworth.

Rolland, J. S. (2005) Cancer and the family: An integrative model. *CANCER Supplement 104*(11) 2584–2589.

Veach, T. A., Nicholas, D. R., & Barton, M. A. (2002) *Cancer and the family life cycle: A practitioner's guide* New York: Brunner-Routledge.

PART 1

LESSONS FROM AND FOR SPECIFIC GROUPS

Helping Parents Understand Cancer in Children and Young Adults: Parents' Guide to Meeting the Educational Needs of Their Child with Cancer

Lena R. Gaddis

W hen your child is first diagnosed with cancer, schooling may not be a priority for you. However, it is generally agreed that returning to school as early as possible is in the best interest of the child. Once you learn the nature of the disease and the course of treatment, you will probably begin to consider how your child might be affected cognitively, academically, and socially by his or her condition, and how to deal with the school in making sure your child's educational needs are met. The purpose of this chapter is to assist you, as parents, in understanding the possible outcomes of the disease, advise you of the legal rights pertaining to your child, and provide you with resources where you can obtain more information regarding the education of your child.

What Outcomes Should I Expect?

Academic Performance

Problems associated with pediatric cancers and treatments may include difficulties in attention, memory, processing speed, planning and organization, writing, copying, learning visual information, performing math calculations, and reading comprehension. Various factors influence the degree of difficulties experienced by children. Children who are younger at onset, girls, and those whose condition involves the brain or the spinal cord may have more problems (Katz & Madan-Swain, 2006). For some children, these difficulties may be evident upon the completion of treatment, but for others they may take some time to appear. You and your school should monitor your child's academic progress so that problems may be identified as early as possible.

Social Outcomes

A child with cancer who returns to school may be viewed as less socially competent, experience feelings of social isolation, and feel rejected by peers. Studies in which children were asked about their emotions found that they experience no more depression or anxiety than children who have not experienced cancer. Interestingly, adolescent survivors of cancer sometimes report having higher self-esteem than other children (Marsland, Ewing, & Thompson, 2006; Fuemmeler, Mullins, & Carpentier, 2006).

How Can I Help My Child Return to School?

Remember that every child is different and may or may not experience the academic and social difficulties noted above. However, you will want to be prepared in the event they do emerge. Below are some strategies that may make your child's return to school easier.

1. Maintain a connection with the school from the beginning of your child's illness with occasional updates to the school principal and teacher. If your child has to miss a significant number of days of school, ask your school about *homebound* services, in which a teacher visits your home and provides instruction and/or tutoring. If your child has an extended hospital stay, the hospital may have an education coordinator who can assist with your child's educational needs.

2. Educate school personnel and classmates about the disease. If your child has been treated at a children's hospital or cancer center, there is often a nurse or other staff member who visits the school to talk to children in your child's class before he or she returns. If this is not the case, you may want to speak to the school nurse to see if someone could assume that role. Children who return to school during or after their illness may experience hair loss, loss or gain of weight, or scars, among other changes in appearance. Students should be prepared for these physical changes in their classmate. Children and adolescents will often have questions and misconceptions about illnesses. For example, younger children may want to know if you can "catch cancer" or if you "get cancer because you are bad." Older children and adolescents may want to know the probability of getting cancer or the scientific basis of the disease. An excellent document called *Learning & Living with Cancer: Advocating for your Child's Educational Needs* is available on the Lance Armstrong Foundation Web site (http://www.livestrong.org). It provides ideas for classroom presentation that could be used by the school nurse or other appropriate individual.

3. Seek accommodations for your child at school, which should help with access to education. For instance, accommodations might include a second set of books for home use, release from a requirement to participate in physical education activities, permission to wear a hat or scarf to school (some schools prohibit this), snacks, and a shortened school day. The Lance Armstrong Foundation Web site mentioned earlier provides excellent rationales for these accommodations that you can provide to your school. Your child may actually have a legal right to accommodations (see discussion of legal issues below).

4. Identify someone at the school as the go-to person to support your child. There is evidence that returning students feel and are viewed as socially isolated. This person could routinely check in with your child, maybe daily in the beginning. Having a trusted individual to turn to for support as he or she reintegrates into the activities of everyday school life may be comforting to your child.

5. Identify a liaison between the medical team and the school to make sure academic and medical needs are achieved. Some children may experience nausea, diarrhea, fatigue, and other symptoms that require special attention from the classroom teacher, the school nurse, and other school personnel. Your child may require rest periods, extra fluids, extra opportunities to use the bathroom, etc. These factors may be best explained by someone from the medical team.

6. Your child may need short-term counseling. There may be a number of issues for which counseling could be helpful. Regarding schooling, counseling may focus on providing strategies for coping with situations faced once he or she returns to school. Your child needs to be prepared for questions that classmates might ask and how they might be answered. Also, your child may need to know when assistance is needed and how to ask for it.

What Legal Rights Does My Child Have?

At first, you may not be comfortable with the idea of your child having a disability (in addition to having cancer), but your child may be entitled to disability-related services that can help him or her be successful in school. There are two pieces of legislation you should be aware of before you enter that discussion.

Section 504 of the Rehabilitation Act of 1973

This is generally referred to as Section 504, or simply 504. It is considered a *civil rights* law that protects both children and adults with disabilities. It states:

No otherwise qualified handicapped individual in the United States . . . shall solely by reason of his handicap, be excluded from participation in, be denied the benefits of, or be subject to discrimination under any activity receiving federal financial assistance. (Rehabilitation Act of 1973, Section 504, 20 U.S.C. § 794(a))

To be eligible for services under Section 504, there must be an identified impairment that substantially limits at least one major life activity. *Substantially limits* is not defined very clearly in the law, but major life activities include walking, seeing, hearing, speaking, breathing, reading, writing, performing math calculations, working, caring for oneself, etc. This is a very broad law that entitles people with disabilities, including children with acute and chronic illnesses such as cancer, to accommodations, modifications, and services, which allows *access to education.*

A school building usually has a 504 team. For school-age children, accommodation, modifications, and services are usually outlined in a *504 plan.* While this plan technically does not have to be in writing, it would be advantageous to request a written document. Some possible accommodations are mentioned above. Others might include a shorter school day, dispensing of medications, and notification of outbreaks of communicable diseases in the school. There are many other possibilities; your child's medical team may have additional suggestions. You can find examples of 504 plans on the Internet. One site that may prove helpful is *specialchildren.about.com.* Enter "section 504" into the site's search engine to view many links on the topic, some of which contain samples of 504 plans.

Individuals with Disabilities Education Act (IDEA)

IDEA was originally put into place in 1975. It is revised every few years and was last revised in 2004. The law requires that every child be provided with a *free and appropriate public education.* The threshold of eligibility is considerably higher than that for Section 504, with your child having to meet specific criteria in order to qualify for services. It also offers the most protection for you and your child because a number of safeguards and protections are attached. Your school should provide you with a document covering parental rights in which these safeguards and protections are explained. One of the rights explained in this document is that you always have a right to challenge the school's actions. IDEA is the most comprehensive law pertaining to the education of children with disabilities, and thus a lot of components and details are contained within it. In order to be a good advocate for your child, you may want to learn more. I have provided some resources in the list below that should assist you in doing this.

The school should provide an evaluation of your child's current standing and review that information at a meeting with you. You may be asked to provide information about your child's development, as well as activities they routinely do at home and in the community. Your child may be administered tests of cognitive, academic, and other abilities.

IDEA requires that parents be a part of the *multidisciplinary team* that will review information and make decisions regarding your child's educational needs. Depending on your child's needs, this team may comprise the classroom teacher, a special education teacher, the school principal, related service providers, a school counselor, a school psychologist, and, if appropriate, your child. At your request, a member of your child's medical team, an advocate, a family member, and/or a friend may be present at meetings regarding your child.

One of the keys to eligibility under this law is that the disability *must affect educational performance*. Like many terms in IDEA, educational performance is not defined, but schools often say that if a child is not making failing grades and is promoted to the next grade, then he or she is not eligible for special education services because educational performance is not affected. However, IDEA clearly states otherwise:

> . . . states must make a free appropriate public education available to 'any individual child with a disability who needs special education and related services, even if the child has not failed or been retained in a course or grade, and is advancing from grade to grade.' [§300.101(c)(1)]

It also has been interpreted that grades and standardized tests alone (this is the type of test your child will likely be administered in the evaluation process described above) should not be the sole basis for determining the affect on educational performance of the child being considered for special education. Rather, a broader view should be taken to include how your child's condition affects social, behavioral, and other domains. Finally, a 1995 letter from the Office of Special Education Programs (a federal governing body), clarified that the multidisciplinary team may consider the extent to which a child has been provided outside learning assistance such as tutoring or extraordinary help from a parent or a teacher, as this may be the reason the child is making passing grades. Such circumstances reflect that the child's current educational performance is a result of the extra help, and not what it might be without this help. Should the issue of educational performance be raised, ask the team to consider all factors pertaining to your child.

If your child receives services under IDEA, an *Individual Education Plan* (IEP) will be developed. The IEP should include, among other components, present levels of performance, measurable goals and objectives, related services as appropriate (things like transportation, speech and language services, and classroom aides), and statement as to the need for an extended school year (when your child requires year-round school in order to maintain skills). This should not be taken to mean that your child would or should receive every available service, but the team should address these and related issues. Typically the IEP is reviewed yearly, but you may ask that the IEP be reviewed any time you believe your child's needs have changed and/or the goals and objectives should be revised.

Individuals ages 3 to 21 are covered by IDEA. Thirteen categories of disability are outlined in this law. The two that may most likely apply to your child are *Other Health Impaired* (OHI) and *Specific Learning Disabilities* (SLD).

Other Health Impaired (OHI). OHI may be the most appropriate designation under IDEA for children with illnesses such as cancer, as it encompasses children with acute and chronic health problems, categories in which cancer is included. A child identified as OHI is one

> . . . having limited strength, vitality or alertness, including a heightened alertness to environmental stimuli, that results in limited alertness with respect to the educational environment, that is due to chronic or acute health problems . . . and adversely affects a child's educational performance. [Individuals with Disabilities Education Improvement Act of 2004, 34 Code of Federal Regulations §300.7(c)(9)]

Federal regulations list examples of conditions, including leukemia, that would warrant an OHI designation. This, however, is not an exhaustive list. Children recovering from other types of cancer would be included. For a child to receive services under OHI, the condition must result in the limitations stated above and must adversely affect educational performance to a degree that special education is necessary for the child to progress through the general curriculum. A medical diagnosis is not sufficient for a student to be identified with a disability under IDEA.

Specific Learning Disability (SLD). This diagnosis may be appropriate if your child has developed academic or processing difficulties as a result of illness and treatment. As indicated above, these problems may not become evident in the early post-treatment period, but rather in later stages, so your child's academic progress should be monitored. The same requirement of adverse effect on educational performance applies to SLD. Federal code defines SLD as

> . . . a disorder in one or more of the basic psychological processes involved in understanding or in using language, spoken or written, which disorder may manifest itself in the imperfect ability to listen, think, speak, read, write, spell, or do mathematical calculations. (Individuals with Disabilities Education Improvement Act of 2004, 20 U.S.C. §1401 [30])

Children with SLD may be provided services in a special education classroom for all or part of the school day. This approach typically offers a smaller student-teacher ratio and more individualized instruction and attention. Another possibility is that your child will stay in his or her regular classroom and receive support services from a special educator; this approach is called *inclusion*. Inclusion allows your child to return to a familiar environment and maintain sustained contact with peers. Some-times the recommended placement for receiving services is influenced by the philosophy of the school district, but you should discuss with your team what would be the most appropriate for your child. Each approach has pros and cons, so do your homework before a placement meeting.

Conclusion

A child who returns to school while recovering from cancer may face many obstacles. However, there are ways to make the transition easier. An involved parent and a supportive school environment are key to the success of this process. The trials you and your family have experienced during your child's cancer have probably taken a toll on you physically and emotionally. Working with your school to ensure the best access to education can be a complicated process that is difficult to maneuver even for parents of healthy children. Do not be afraid to ask for help from family members, friends, or an experienced advocate should the process become overwhelming! The resources and references listed below should also help.

Resources

* American Cancer Society. *Children diagnosed with cancer: Returning to school.* Available at http://www.cancer.org/docroot/CRI/content/CRI_2_6x_When_Your_Child_Goes_Back_to_School.asp. Information at this site includes strategies for maintaining communication with the school, expectations for your child's school performance, and gaining services for your child.
* Lance Armstrong Foundation. *Learning and living with cancer: Advocating for your child's educational needs.* Available at http://www.live strong.org/site/c.khLXK1PxHmF/b.2662109/. This document outlines strategies for transitioning your child back to school and acquiring needed educational services.
* Wrightslaw. Available at http://www.wrightslaw.com/. This site contains a tremendous amount of information regarding legal issues that may pertain to your child's educational needs. The site is maintained by attorneys, but it is not written in technical language. On the home page, in the menu to the left is a list of topics that link to information about Section 504 and IDEA, as well as other relevant topics.

References

Fuemmeler, B. F., Mullins, L. L., & Carpentier, M. Y. (2006). Peer, friendship issues, and emotional well being. In R. T. Brown (Ed.), *Comprehensive handbook of childhood cancer and sickle cell disease: A biopsychological approach* (pp. 100–118). New York: Oxford Press.

Individuals with Disabilities Education Improvement Act of 2004, H.R.1350 Public Law108–446 (2004).

Katz, E. R., & Madan-Swain, A. (2006). Maximizing school, academic, and social outcomes in children and adolescents with cancer. In R. T. Brown (Ed.), *Comprehensive handbook of childhood cancer and sickle cell disease: A biopsychological approach* (pp. 313–338). New York: Oxford Press.

Marsland, A. L., Ewing, L. J., & Thompson, A. (2006). Psychological and social effects of surviving childhood cancer. In R. T. Brown (Ed.), *Comprehensive handbook of childhood cancer and sickle cell disease: A biopsychological approach* (pp. 237–261). New York: Oxford Press.

Rehabilitation Act of 1973, Section 504, 29 U.S.C. Sec. 794 Public Law 93–112 (1973).

CHAPTER 4

Helping Children and Young Adults Understand Parental Cancer

Mika Niemelä and Leena Väisänen

A parent's serious illness will be reflected in the life of the entire family—serious illness can affect that person's ability to act as a parent. There have been numerous research reports on the effects of a parent's serious illness on communication between family members, day-to-day life, and parents' ability to meet the demands of their children. Regarding cancer diseases, recent research has shown that tailored, child-centered methods are recommended for helping families cope when a parent is seriously ill. In this chapter, we share our experience in conducting family interventions when a parent is diagnosed with cancer. We begin by describing how children might respond to a parent's serious illness. We then offer suggestions on how parents can help, and conclude with a case example demonstrating our family intervention.

The children of a parent suffering from cancer may react to the changed situation of the family with various behavioral and emotional problems (see chapter 2). Although unable to comprehend the concept of illness, an infant will react instinctively to changes in a parent's behavior, as well as to changes in environment and daily routines. By preschool age, a child will understand if the parent's condition is said to be terminal. Children cry, become afraid, and are emotionally shocked when they realize that a parent is ill. They, too, may suffer from somatic symptoms such as headaches and have difficulty falling asleep at night.

Those of school age may become involved in more arguments with peers and have difficulties in controlling their level of intimacy with the parent who is ill. They experience loneliness, they often cry, and they feel unloved. They say that they are sad, unhappy, and depressed. Difficulties are more likely to occur for a child of school age if the family is small, or if the child is the oldest sibling or is an only child. The physical limitations affecting a parent are especially difficult for girls. Children of school age may also suffer from headaches and sleeping difficulties.

Adolescents are able to verbalize the effects and implications of a parent's illness, yet may have strong reactions, such as excessive risk behavior. In addition, they often have to take care of younger siblings; as a result, such adolescents may have difficulties fulfilling their own obligations regarding schoolwork, for example. They may suffer from emotional symptoms such as anxiety and depression in response to the parent's decreased physical abilities. Adolescent girls, especially, may suffer from somatic symptoms such as headache, abdominal pains, dizziness, sleeping disorders, and lack of appetite.

How to Help Children at Home

The protective factors in children's lives are known from research. They are good relationships with parents, one or more good friends, regular school attendance, hobbies, and relationships with trustworthy adults. One of the most important factors is that a child should understand what it means when a parent has cancer. This knowledge will help the child to carry on.

You are the best expert to tell your children about your cancer. Start when you feel safe and know what to say. You have to decide when the time is right to tell them. Tell about what your cancer is, how it is treated, what the purpose of the treatment is, and what the side effects are. Suggest that your children ask questions and tell you how they are feeling.

Children find different ways of coping, and it is only through dialogue that you can discover these. Talking together increases cooperation and communication within a family. You cannot have all the answers that children need, but you can do your best in an honest manner. Sometimes children don't have questions, or they don't want to say any more. Talk can serve as an opening and make it easier for children to speak about it later, at any time, when they have questions. It is also possible to take your child to the hospital to see how you are being treated, and to arrange a discussion with an oncologist or nurse.

Children become stronger emotionally when they learn to face difficult things with support from their parents. They know it is possible to survive and lead a normal childhood in spite of a parent's cancer. The three most common things that children are afraid of are:

1. Did I cause the cancer?
2. Will it be transmitted to me?
3. Is my parent dying, so that I'll be left alone?

If you want to check on how your children are doing, it may be a good idea to map out the different fields in their lives:

1. Ask your children what they are doing at school, and tell the teachers or other significant contact persons at the school about your illness. Explain how you and your child want this changed family situation to be taken into account regarding your child. For instance, it also would be good if you can describe your child's way of reacting to your illness, so that misunderstandings at school will be more easily avoided. In one case, for example, the parents had a discussion with their seven-year-old girl; she said that she sometimes remembered her mother's situation and became sad while in class. She said it was hard to hide her tears from the others. Almost all the other pupils in her class knew about her mother's illness, but she didn't want to cry among them. So the parents made a deal with the teacher and the school nurse that if she became sad she could go to the school nurse. This arrangement was a small thing, but quite a relief for that little girl.
2. Ask how your children are getting on with their friends, and whether they have told their friends about your illness. Every family has its own way of talking about these things. A big secret is hard to keep, and openness is usually a better course. It is also difficult for a child to make excuses to friends if the friends can't be told the real situation. Ask directly whether there is any bullying at the school or among the other children. If there is, intervene in the situation or ask for help in such an intervention. Bullying is always a matter for adults.
3. It is also important to take an interest in children's hobbies and daily routines. Because of your illness, you may not be able to take part in those things as before, but it is important to stand by your child. It may be that someone close to him or her can take care of these things. A trusted adult from outside the family is an important protective factor for children. If there is someone who can move into your home while you are in the hospital, for example, this could be an appropriate thing to do. If you need extra help from social or health services, for instance, it is important that it is always the same people who visit your home. New faces every day are not good for making an environment that feels safe for children.

Serious illness in a parent is always a huge change for the whole family. One father said that it was like the family facing a tsunami on their own. In the case of an overwhelming life situation such as cancer, doing little things for the children means great things for the future. As one parent said, when there seems that there is no future, it is actually the children that are the future!

Preventative Family Intervention and Cancer

Preventative family intervention, as originally created by Professor William Beardslee of Harvard University, was used in working with parents who had clinical depression. Beginning in 2001, Beardslee's intervention was used as part of The Effective Family Project led by Professor Tytti Solantaus at Finland's National Institute for Health and Welfare. It also was aimed at providing support and prevention for families with a depressed parent. Our work at Oulu University Hospital in Finland has involved adapting the preventative family intervention for use when a parent is diagnosed with cancer. In 2003, a partnership began between the hospital's cancer units and its Department of Psychiatry, where we are based, and where we carry out the family intervention. Parents have been satisfied with our process and outcomes. Our aim and hope is that in the future, all families who desire it should be provided with family intervention.

The family intervention consists of five to eight family sessions. The parents are first interviewed, and future sessions with their children are planned. Next, each child in the family is interviewed separately. The parents are given reports on the sessions with children. The parents assist in planning a session where all family members will be together. Topics addressed in the "all family" session include:

1. the well-being of the children,
2. communication between the family members,
3. information regarding illness, and
4. protective factors for the child.

These topics may be addressed in follow-up sessions as needed.

Case Example: The Virtanen Family

Sofia was a patient in the oncology unit and was asked there if she had any children and if she wanted to talk about them. Sofia thought this was a good idea, so a nurse from the oncology unit called the Department of Psychiatry to arrange our meeting with Sofia and her husband, Martti. We told the couple about our family intervention, explaining its structure and content (see previous section). The parents thought it was worth trying, and we agreed that if they had second thoughts, or if it proved to be different from what they were expecting, we would pause or stop the intervention. After the first session, both parents said they wanted to continue the intervention. Sofia said that she regarded cancer as a serious chronic illness that she had to live with for the rest of her life.

The First Session with Parents. Sofia and Martti have three children: a 16-year-old daughter and two sons, ages 19 and 13. Sofia's first breast cancer diagnosis was made in the early 1990s, when their eldest child was only two years old. This diagnosis was a shock; their family life was still in an early phase (see chapter 2). Martti explained that they just had built a new house and that he had started his first permanent job. He remembered how he thought his wife was going to die. He just remembered walking down a long hospital corridor carrying his son in his arms. It was like walking in a fog. Sofia agreed that *fog* was a good word to describe their feelings at that time.

The couple were greatly relieved to hear the doctor say that surgical treatment would be enough and were further relieved to hear that the tumor had been totally removed. Thus, after a few follow-up visits, Sofia was declared to be cured. The couple's confidence in the future grew. As the years went by, their two younger children were born. They said that during that time they no longer thought of cancer.

In 2001, Sofia felt tired. She went to the health center and after various tests was referred to the oncology unit of Oulu University Hospital. A different kind of tumor was found this time. She said she didn't know whether it was a metastasis of the earlier breast cancer or a new tumor. After surgical treatment and radiation therapy, she had quite a long period off work. She was at home trying to get back on her feet and trying to take care of their three children. Martti and Sofia described how they felt the same cold fog come over them again, even thicker and colder than before. They felt fear all the time, and sometimes a light glimmer of hope, depending on the news they received at follow-up visits. It was a roller coaster of hope and fear, said Martti.

In 2005, Sofia again felt unwell. Again she went to the health center, was given tests, and was referred to the oncology unit. Once again the news was not good—several metastases were found in her lungs. She received intensive chemotherapy. In 2008, at the time of our family intervention session, Sofia was still under treatment.

The Second Session with Parents. One week after the first session, Sofia and Martti came for a second parents' session. They said that the week since the first meeting had gone well, and they were ready to continue the intervention. Sofia added that the previous week's conversation had been hard and that many things had come into her mind afterward— from the days when the children were little—but everything felt good.

We summarized the things that had been talked about during the first session. The parents were asked to identify if anything had been misunderstood. We explained that the purpose of this second session was to discuss their children, and that if they decided to allow us to meet their children, they would help us in deciding what concerns to address with the children.

Sofia and Martti said first that their eldest son, Petri (age 19), was now doing better than previously—he had had a lot of trouble at school, especially elementary school. During that time, the teacher had called home to say that Petri was in fights with other boys; sometimes he didn't want to go to school. He had now just qualified as a plumber and was looking for work and a place of his own in which to live. He wanted to be independent; he didn't want to live at home any longer and accept money from his parents. Sofia and Martti supported his desire to be independent, but they were worried about the loneliness they saw in their son. They said that he had only a few friends and that he did not speak about any personal matters at home. They said they understood that Petri was a young man and that it was quite normal not to speak about his own affairs with his parents, but his silence had lasted for a long time. Both parents thought it would be a good idea to invite Petri to participate in their children's individual sessions. Sofia and Martti hoped that Petri would share his worries and personal matters in the individual session with us and subsequently share his thoughts also with them. Sofia added that there was a time when she was very afraid of death, and she thought that Petri may have seen her fear. Sofia thought that all the children should be asked about any fears of her death.

The parents described their 16-year-old daughter, Jaana, as very different from Petri. She had a lot of friends and was very athletic, coming and going all the time. She was in school and doing fine. However, Sofia and Martti felt that because Jaana was so busy, they were unsure how she was really coping. They agreed that she should be asked about this.

Sofia and Martti reported that Sami, their 13-year-old son, was doing fine at school. Like his sister, he had many friends, and he spent his time playing soccer. They described him as a strong person who persisted in things once he had made up his mind. In many ways he was like Jaana—staying busy, for instance. The parents thought he should be asked what he said to his friends about his mother's situation. One thing was obvious to them—he did not want his mother to be seen by his friends during her chemotherapy. When she had lost her hair, he would always run up with the wig, saying "Put this on—put this on" when he saw his friends coming to the house.

Individual Sessions with the Children. Jaana **(age 16)** was the first to come for a meeting. She was a vivacious young girl. She said that her mother had told her what this was all about—that the session was a kind of assessment of how the children were coping with their mother's illness. She said that her mother had been ill all the time that she could remember. The most difficult times were when her mother was in the hospital, sick from the chemotherapy. Jaana had always been afraid that her mother was going to die in the hospital; it was always a relief when her mother came home. The enormous worries in her parents' life made her keep her own worries to herself. She didn't want to disturb her parents.

Jaana said she felt that there was a place inside her where she was all alone—and this was a lonely place. When asked to explain, she gave this example: "Before a lesson starts at school, all of the students chat. But if you have your own pressing thoughts, including your mother's illness, a fear of death, and so on, you feel cut off from the others." Now, she felt that she could tell some of her friends about how she felt, and she received support from her nearest friends, but her mother's illness was not a subject to talk to everyone about. She found Sami was very close to her, but Petri was more distant. She didn't know why, but it had always been like that.

Petri **(age 19)**. Petri came for his meeting in the afternoon on the same day we met with Jaana. His parents had been uncertain as to whether he would come at all. However, Petri said that he had decided to come because his father had told him that he would not be forced to do anything and that he could talk only if he wanted. We confirmed this, and Petri proceeded to talk a lot about his current life. He said he was happy that school was finally over and that he was anxious to go out to work and earn his own money. On being told that his parents thought he wanted to be independent, Petri smiled and said that it was true.

Petri confirmed that he had only a few friends, and that there was only one with whom he could share personal matters like his mother's illness. They spent their time tuning their cars and driving around the town. He said that he had never had any friends at school. He confirmed that he often felt lonely. Asked whether he chose to be alone or was left alone by others, he said that both were true. At first there had been fights with some boys during breaks at school, and later he had suffered from teasing and bullying. He thought it might be some kind of role he had acquired during the first years at school that had remained with him. He said it was too late do to anything now, but gave us permission to discuss this with his parents. He, however, didn't want talk about his situation with the whole family.

Petri said he would prefer to talk with his father alone, but hoped that his father would start the conversation. He had never wanted to tell anyone at home about the bullying for fear of worrying his parents. He declined the offer of therapy for this. He had been most worried about his mother's situation at the time of the second cancer diagnosis, when she had been vomiting and had to be taken to the hospital by ambulance. The fear that she might die had been in his mind then, but not anymore. He wanted to know about possible phases of his mother's illness, however, and also about her current situation

Sami **(age 13)**. Sami came with his mother, who sat and waited in the lobby. Sami was slightly nervous when he sat down. When, to lighten the beginning of the conversation, he was told that his parents had described him as a magnificent soccer player, he smiled wryly. After quite a long soccer conversation, the topic turned to his school and friends. School was okay, and he liked sports most of all. He had four or five close friends, and many others, too, with whom he spent some time. Sami said he was close to his parents and that if he had worries, he would tell his mother. He said Jaana was very close to him, and he would sometimes help Petri fix his car. Sami wanted to know how his mother was doing.

The Third Session with Parents: Planning Family Meeting. Sofia and Martti said that Jaana had told them all about her session. Sofia was happy, saying that she felt relieved and had heard for the first time about some of the things that Janna had experienced—they stayed up late at night talking after Jaana's individual meeting. In contrast, both sons merely reported that their parents would hear everything in their own meeting.

We told the parents that we felt they had wonderful children and that it was a privilege to work with them. (This was not just a pleasantry, as such things are not said in the Finnish culture unless they are really meant.) The discussion then went on to the main topics raised with the children and to a review of the protective factors for the children that existed in their family. Sofia and Martti were very emotional when they heard Petri's story. They said they knew something about the bullying and that they had had meetings with his teachers and so on, but they didn't know that it never ended completely. Martti said that they would discuss it with him that evening.

In planning for a family meeting with everyone present, the parents identified two main topics. Sofia wanted to tell everyone the whole story of her illness, from the beginning to the present day, and to explain what she knew about the future. She said it was better for the children to know the facts so that they could prepare themselves if there was still a need for hospital treatment, etc. The second topic was communication to the children that they should bring all their worries to their parents if they needed to. It would not make their mother's illness any worse, and their father would be able to do something to help them. An appointment was made for a home visit. It is possible to meet families either at the hospital clinic or at home, but many clinicians prefer family meetings at home.

The Family Meeting. The Virtanens' home is located in the beautiful countryside near the sea, about 30 minutes from our office at University Hospital. The family was waiting in their large living room, which had a huge dining table and impressive rural-style furniture. The meeting began with a summary of their progress, briefly describing the first two meetings with the parents and then those with the children, followed by the third meeting with the mother and father to plan what to discuss at the family meeting. It was explained that the parents had decided to speak about two topics, and that it was the mother who wanted to start.

There was a moment of silence before Sofia began: "Petri was only little when I was taken ill for the first time. We were building this house." She then told her cancer story, up to the current moment. She asked the children whether, for instance, they remembered visiting her in the hospital—the children, mostly Jaana, commented briefly or filled in some details. Sofia cried a little, especially when she remembered the moments when she was away and the children had to come home from school alone, and she was especially sorry for Petri, who was a little school-aged boy at that time. She also said she hoped that the children knew that they were the whole world for her and that there was nothing to compare with them.

Sofia also told the children that her cancer would never be cured entirely—she would have to take medication for the rest of her life. At the moment, everything seemed to be all right, but she had to visit the doctor frequently. If there were any changes, she promised to tell the children.

Next, Martti began by saying that the children could tell their mother and father anything—any of their worries and concerns—and that their mother would not get worse if they told her things about their lives. He went on to say how hard it had been for everyone in the family in the past years, but emphasized, again, that there was no need for the children to spare their parents worries or bad news.

The entire conversation was held among the family members. The parents asked if there was anything more the children wanted to know, and they answered the children's questions.

Follow-Up Session. One month after the family meeting, Sofia and Martti reported that it was easier to breathe at home. (This meeting was held only with parents; however, it is possible to include the whole family in a follow-up session.) Sofia and Martti were happy that they had asked for the family intervention. Petri was working at his first job, although they were still worried about his loneliness. Martti checked on him now and then, asking him how he was doing. Jaana was doing fine, as before, and Sofia was enjoying good conversations with her. Sami was the same as ever, but they could now laugh together and remember how busy he had been at one time, making sure Sofia wore her wig when his friends were over.

Conclusion

In our family intervention, it is central to observe the children's situation and discuss these observations with the parents. Concentrating on children in a family dealing with cancer is seen as helping the parents, too—they can analyze their own concerns for their children. As it is important for the family intervention to be based on knowledge of factors protecting children, these factors give the parents an opportunity to observe their children's coping in more detail.

Research has been conducted in Oulu (Niemelä, Väisänen, Marshall, Hakko & Räsänen, in press) recording the experiences of health care workers engaging children with a parent who has cancer. Seven research participants described in interviews the experiences they had had in child-centered work by recalling cases with such families. They described how the work with the children had led them to reevaluate their own work—previously focused only on adults—and how it had become impossible for them to work solely with individuals and adults. They felt that issues were brought to light by listening to the children who might otherwise have remained unnoticed. It was especially important, they agreed, to listen to the situation of children who were on the threshold of puberty. Their worries and concerns seemed to remain more hidden than those of the younger children, who expressed their thoughts more readily. This observation is an interesting one because it is known that adolescents, especially girls, suffer from psychological and somatic symptoms if a parent is ill.

According to the team's experiences, even just listening to the children alleviated their concerns. Conversations between family members, either at home or together with a worker at a joint family session, were beneficial in opening up discussions about an unresolved situation. As a result, the parents themselves were often put at ease. Parents who are extremely concerned over their children have a hard time talking about anything regarding the future—a discussion "stalls" due to the anxiety caused by the illness whenever the discussion moves to the matters of the future.

The object of family intervention is dialogue among family members. A dialogue-based approach, together with a completely voluntary basis for the work, provides it with strength and appeal. For instance, while a psychiatrist was a participant in the family meeting of the Virtanen family case example, the psychiatrist did not direct the meeting. Our role in facilitating the family intervention is to enable a new kind of discussion to take place, but it is the parents who lead the discussion.

Reference

Niemelä, M., Väisänen, L., Marshall, C.A., Hakko, H., & Räsänen, S. (in press). The experiences of mental health professionals utilizing structured child and family-centered interventions in families with parental cancer. *CANCER NURSING: An International Journal for Cancer Care.*

Coping in an African American Family

CHAPTER 5

A Daughter's Acceptance

Deirdre Cobb-Roberts

I can do all things through him who strengthens me.

Philippians 4:13, *The Bible,*
King James Version

This narrative represents my emotional, spiritual, and ongoing journey. I am reminded of a scripture from *The Bible*: "To whom much is given, much is required" (Luke 12:48). This has become my mantra. I repeat this mantra daily just to make it to the next doctor's appointment, kid's football game, manuscript deadline, or disagreement with Mom. My journey has been paved with an abundance of support both formal and informal, and I hope my story of coping with cancer in an African American family can lessen the load of others faced with this challenge and opportunity.

Over the last two years, I have prayed constantly (although I soon realized my prayers were not specific enough), consulted formal research on anal cancer with metastasis, attended support groups, and depended on doctors and friends to provide the educational and emotional support I have needed as a co-survivor. I have learned it was okay to have bad days and days when I questioned why me, and what about me, and the divinity of coincidence. Coping has been critical because I am not only a daughter, but also a caregiver. We moved Mom to be near me in March

2007 to continue her cancer treatment—I had to balance that new responsibility with family and work life.

It's 2009, and Mom is still with us and fighting cancer every day. We have been through surgeries, challenges to independence, mother-daughter battles, failed treatment trials, and now hospice. Each day is a gift from God, and the most coincidental aspect of all is that Mom and I have been given the opportunity to rediscover our relationship, a potentially lost opportunity if not for her illness. I have constantly asked what lesson I am to take away from this experience, why this valley is important, and the answer is simple: acceptance and patience. "Accept the things you cannot change, change the things that you can, and have the wisdom to know the difference." I am learning to accept God's plan for my mother's life, for mine, and the intersection of both.

When my mother first told me she thought she might have cancer, I immediately went into my positive-thinking mode and said, "No, it has to be something else." In December 2006, it wasn't something else; it was cancer—the big "C." Cancer had finally hit home. For years I had had conversations with friends and colleagues concerning the rapid increase of cancer diagnoses, but until five years ago, cancer was never close to me. My grandmother is a uterine cancer survivor; her sister died of breast cancer. Indeed, a host of distant relatives, friends, and colleagues had cancer, were survivors, or their bodies had been ravaged by the disease. Still, my mother's diagnosis was a real shock. I was unprepared.

In my grandmother's case, we were very concerned. She was 78, and the doctor wanted to perform a hysterectomy. She was not contemplating children at her age, so that was not a concern. However, the thought of major surgery at her age was overwhelming. She lived in Washington, DC, was a committed and devoted member of her church, and had a host of family and friends to support her. My mother, her only child, and I, her only grandchild, were right there by her side before, during, and after surgery. Our being there was expected and what we wanted to do. At the time, I was in graduate school and found my schedule flexible enough to be with her—my grandmother and the matriarch of the family. That was 15 years ago; December 2006 was incredibly different.

How do we support loved ones battling cancer? How do we advocate for our loved ones without stripping them of independence? How do we balance our personal and professional lives? How do we care for ourselves when we are the caregiver? How do we remove the guilt associated with the days when we would rather be doing anything else besides sitting in a doctor's office with a loved one? The answers to these questions are, simply, prayer, support networks, and education. This reflection is of my personal journey as a daughter, mother, wife, colleague, and co-survivor.

As a caregiver and a co-survivor, it was imperative that I educate myself immediately. Of course I "knew" what cancer was in a generic sense, but I now needed to know what we could do about my mother's cancer, to help her, to save her. The first place I consulted was the American Cancer Society as I began my journey of denial, pain, and support. *Cancer Facts & Figures for African Americans 2009–2010* (2009) states that according to the American Cancer Society, "African Americans have the highest death rate and shortest survival of any racial and ethnic group in the U.S. for most cancers" (p. 1). That was a debilitating blow. In my effort to be forearmed with an abundance of information that would help my mother, I was faced with the fact that her fate was already determined, according to the research. In fact, upon further reading I learned that her form of cancer is the third most common cancer in both African American men and women (p. 10). Researchers had identified potential risk factors that increased the likelihood of cancer—but that wasn't us.

My mother went to the doctor regularly, didn't she? She was considered educated and middle-class. This combination should have meant she had access to medical insurance and decent health care benefits, right? She was physically active and very conscious of her weight, so that should have precluded another risk factor, right? She was a smoker, but tobacco use was not an indicator for her form of cancer. So my questions came: Why Mom? Why this? Why now? What will we do? Sadly, my final question seemed to be the most selfish of all—why me? I cannot do this.

Beginning Treatment

Know that I am with you and will keep you wherever you go.

Genesis 28:15

Now a mother, wife, and faculty member, my life was quite different and my responsibilities far greater than when my grandmother was diagnosed with cancer. But Mom was sick—I was all she had. She lived in Chicago, I in Tampa. Mom had no husband, and Grandma was now 90 years old. It was all up to me to provide the emotional support she would need to fight this debilitating, often disabling disease. This would prove challenging—not only her illness, but my situation of being a support person, caregiver, daughter, mother, wife, and professional who lived many miles away. My mother—a loving, strong, intelligent, opinionated, and **independent** African American woman—was facing the biggest battle of her life.

Many will say cancer should not be given that much power, but it's not just the disease itself; there would also be the residual effects of cancer. Chemotherapy, radiation, doctor visits, denial, medication, pain, depression, resentment, distrust, self-pity, change in living environment, and loss of independence would become the additional consequences of cancer. Of course, having cancer was a battle for her, for us; but the loss of independence, her independence as an African American woman, has been the real challenge. There were few places that focused on that particular loss.

The loss of independence for a strong African American woman is often akin to a spiritual death sentence. The African American woman who internalizes her challenges faces real death; she must also face the perceived "death" she believes will fall upon those she trusts with her admission that she needs help. Villarosa (1994) eloquently discusses how being "saddled with the heavy burden of being 'strong' Black women, we have all too often sacrificed our physical, spiritual, and emotional health for the well being of others" (p. 367). This was the burden my mother felt she needed to carry—alone. She felt the need to shield me from the truth, to constantly tell me that everything was going to be fine. She would constantly repeat in our daily conversations that "there is no need to come to Tampa for treatment; I will be fine right here in Chicago, no need to disrupt your life. After all, I am your mother and it is my job to protect you." What she did not understand, nor I at that particular time, was that I needed to be a part of this process. I needed to be there for her, and I needed to be there for me. We needed to be there for each other.

Her treatments began in February 2007, in Chicago. Of course, Mom felt it unnecessary for me to be there during her first round of chemo, but I would not hear of it. I happily arranged for a guest speaker/colleague to cover teaching my class at the university. I made the necessary arrangements for my young children—drop-off, pick-up, after-school sports, and activities. I cooked enough food to cover the week for my husband and kids, and finally, I was headed home, a place I left at 18 years of age. I arrived on a Friday evening. Mom and I went to dinner and spent some quality time catching up; it was like a girls' weekend. Only in the back of my mind, and I am sure in my mother's as well, this weekend was the beginning to an unknown journey. Then it was Monday, and treatments began.

We drove to the hospital. She checked in. I met the doctor and asked him my list of questions. He answered and commended me on the research I had done for my mother's treatment. It was important to me that the doctor viewed me as a partner in my mother's health care, even if she had limited my access. In her opinion, I was there as a courtesy she extended to me—one that required her permission. I was "fairly" comfortable in this subordinate role—such was typically the case in our mother-daughter relationship, even though I was now an adult with a family of my own. However, the doctor provided an insight that was invaluable and empowering. As we discussed my mother's diagnosis and treatment plan, he asked me a series of questions related to culture. He was interested in our religious background, our view of family, and how we made decisions.

It was clear that culture, *our* culture and beliefs, mattered to him in this process. That was a unique and welcomed approach. Silk (2008) contends, "as patients and physicians are expected to partner and corroborate in their care, an understanding of cultural background is even more vital for a physician" (p. 323). The doctor's acknowledgment of our belief system was evidence that he saw my mother as an individual, and that her beliefs might impact her health care decisions. Stage III rectal cancer left Mom with very few options and decisions. Chemotherapy and radiation—surgery was out. The tumor was too large, too advanced.

Once situated in the chemo room, we both took a moment to absorb our surroundings—a single chemo chair/recliner, a second recliner for a guest, a television, and a sink. The room was sterile, quiet, and cold. We got settled and Mom received her meds: the anti-nausea medicine, some fluids, as she was a bit dehydrated, and then her chemotherapy (5-FU plus mitomycin), a four-hour drip. Afterward, we left one facility to head to the next location for radiation. It had been determined that her stage III cancer needed to be treated aggressively, and it was.

The first week consisted of four days of chemo and five days of radiation, and I was there every day. We laughed, ate, and talked, a lot, but never about the cancer and its potential residual effects. Aside from being a bit tired, Mom had tolerated her first week very well—no nausea, and her appetite was decent. She was pleased; I was pleased. I stayed through the weekend, returning home on Sunday and feeling satisfied that this would be smooth sailing; after all, Mom had assured me of such. I had the doctor's promise that Mom would be fine with my returning home. He told me, "Your mom is a strong woman; she is a fighter. She will endure, and we will look after her." His comments were a nice gesture, but he did not really know my mom. How could he be so sure? I was more comfortable knowing that my cousin and two dearest friends (one of whom had lost her mother to brain cancer) were there to stand in for me in my absence. I could leave in peace, right? I did my research, asked questions, supported Mom her first week, and left her in good hands. What else could be done, should be done? I had done what family was supposed to do—"be there." However, there was still something nagging me that I was unable to identify.

The commitment to family is strong within the African American community. In his seminal work, Hill (1971) identified five strengths that were considered primary to the successful functioning and maintenance of the African American family. Those five strengths were strong kinship bond, strong work orientation, adaptability of family roles, strong achievement orientation, and strong religious orientation. Hill (1971, 1999) and others (Boyd-Franklin, 2003; Perkins-Dock, 2005; Bell-Tolliver, Burgess, & Brock, 2009) believed these strengths were the key dispelling the pathologizing theories surrounding the decline of strong and supportive African American families. Our family embodied those strengths and more; we had what it took to get past this and back to normal.

Strong, committed support appeared during the second week of Mom's treatment journey in the form of a mother's love. I was unable to return to Chicago for the next step, and Mom assured me she was fine and needed no support. However, her resolve was challenged when our matriarch, my grandmother, decided it was time to make her appearance. At the age of 90, in her quiet, humble, committed Christian way, she flew from Baltimore from Chicago to see about her baby, her only child. My reports that Mom was doing well and had managed effortlessly the first week fell on deaf ears; she needed to "see" for herself. She needed not only to pray for my mother but to be there to pray with her, and to see her through this challenging period. I knew then what had been tugging at my conscience: true, deliberate, specific, and focused prayer—acknowledgement of fully embracing the notion of letting go and trusting God—a return to my spiritual roots that had been nurtured by my parents, but sustained and constantly demonstrated by my grandparents, especially my grandmothers, two strong African American women.

An Opportunity to Give Back

To whom much is given, much is required.

Luke 12:48

I have always known that I come from a long line of strong African American women, unwavering in all things that are just. The end of Mom's second week of treatment gave me the opportunity to demonstrate that passionate commitment to doing what was right, unconditionally. At the end of the second week, Mom had a terrible reaction to her treatments; she ended up in the intensive care unit for over a week. One of my "sister" friends had gone by to check on Mom in my absence, as she often did. She was a social worker, and her mother had lost her battle to brain cancer a few years earlier, so she possessed a unique awareness of people dealing with cancer and health care in general. She had also known Mom since we were seven years of age. She immediately felt that Mom needed to be seen by her doctor, so she took her to her primary care physician, who immediately sent her to the emergency room. Mom was admitted to the hospital, Grandma was still at the house, in the wintertime, 90 years old, unable to drive, and I was in Tampa, feeling totally helpless and guilty. I should have been there.

Until that precise moment in time, I had taken my wonderfully blessed life for granted. I had attended private school, an academy high school, and a prestigious undergraduate institution, had earned my doctorate, and had a great job, wonderful children, a phenomenal husband, and a host of friends and relatives. I lived in suburban America, my children attended private school, I had cultivated a positive professional reputation, and I had a few extra dollars in the bank for a rainy day, a college plan for the boys, and a retirement plan. Life was grand, wasn't it? I was thankful for all my blessings, wasn't I? I didn't deserve the "burden" of an ailing parent, did I? Life was too good to be interrupted by a parental death. In that precise moment, a scripture came to me: "To whom much is given, much is required."

In an instant, I knew that I had been given much and that now much would be required of me. Could I handle what was required? I never stopped to ponder this question because as soon as I heard Mom was in ICU, nothing else mattered. I was on the next plane back to Chicago. I was going home to give back to a woman who had given so much in her own unique way. I was going home to change roles. I was going home as an adult woman for the first time. I was going home to bring my mother back to Tampa to be here with me. I had come to know and fully respect the power of prayer.

Family Matters

> My mouth shall speak of wisdom; and the meditation of my heart shall be of understanding.
>
> Psalm 49:3

Once back in Chicago, I went immediately to the hospital and assured Mom that we would get through this together, and that I would handle everything. I met with doctors to ascertain what had gone wrong; they merely offered that Mom had had a negative reaction to the treatment— not acceptable to my way of thinking. By now, I had been in touch with patient relations at the cancer center on my university's campus. A friend of a friend assured me that if Mom got a referral to the center, she would be sure to get her in to see an oncologist immediately. Now the only problem was Mom's insurance—an HMO. I prayed that God would order my steps and direct me toward the path of least resistance. I located Mom's insurance papers and made a series of phone calls. Every call was met with an open attitude and a wealth of information on what I needed to do in order to transfer her insurance to Tampa for use at the H. Lee Moffitt Cancer Center and Research Institute, a National Cancer Institute comprehensive cancer center. It could not get any better than this, right? Actually, it got worse—not for Mom, but for our family, my husband in particular.

In this story I have neglected the story of my husband's simultaneous journey. At the very point at which I needed to fly home to be with

Mom, my husband was at his family home in Urbana, Illinois, with his father, who was dying from cancer. I will never forget his words when I called to discuss Mom's situation: "I will come home to be with the boys so that you can go be with your mom, because you have a chance to save your mom. Dad is past the point of saving, and I have had the pleasure of being with him through what your mom is beginning to experience." I appreciated his unselfish commitment to me and family in a broader sense. He traveled back to Florida so that I could leave.

While in Chicago with Mom, I received a call that my father-in-law was in the "active stages of death," a hospice term. I and a girlfriend drove two hours south to Urbana in a winter storm so that I could say good-bye for both myself and my husband. Mom was released from the hospital on February 26, 2007; we both flew to Tampa on March 2, 2007; and my father-in-law passed on March 7, 2007. George Riley, you are missed and forever loved.

Learning the Meaning of Coincidence

> And we know that all things work together for good to them that
> love God, to them who are called according to His purpose.
>
> Romans 8:28

Turner (2008) uses the terms "God allowed" or "God arranged" in discussing coincidence: "Many folks often use this term to speak of event occurrences that they believe to be accidental or pure luck. What most don't know is that 'coincide,' the root form of coincidence is a mathematical term that means to 'correspond exactly' or 'align perfectly'" (p.11). I have experienced several such coincidences along this journey, the first being my birth to my parents, who divorced several years ago. Their desire for me to pursue an advanced degree led me to the path of a career in higher education, and eventually to interview for a job at a university that was home to one of the top cancer centers and research institutes in the country. The friendships I formed early in life and later in my adult life would be the ones I would learn to lean on, and these friends would anticipate my needs before I even made a request of them, everything from getting Mom to dialysis, to picking up my children when I was unable, to helping my mother unpack while I was teaching my class.

My father's wife, my other mother, has been unconditional in her support. My children have learned a sense of compassion and family commitment that I never could have taught them, especially being in a city where we have no biological family. Still, we have met a family that believes in adoption, and they have adopted us, thus demonstrating that family is defined not only by blood, but also by relationships. My husband's loss has taught me patience with my mother as I live with his pain of losing his dad; he constantly reminds me: "Do all that you can with and for your mom because she is still here. Don't worry about us because we are fine." A final note of thanks for the coincidence of my birth goes to my father, the wind beneath my wings, who taught me the value of never giving up.

References

American Cancer Society. (2009). *Cancer facts & figures for African Americans 2009–2010.*

Bell-Tolliver, L., Burgess, R., & Brock, L. J. (2009). African American therapists working with African American families: An exploration of the strengths perspective in treatment. *Journal of Marriage and Therapy, 35*(3), 293–307.

Boyd-Franklin, N. (2003). *Black families in therapy.* New York: Guilford Press.

Hill, R. B. (1971). *The strengths of Black families.* New York: Emerson Hall.

Hill, R. B. (1999). *The strengths of African American families: Twenty-five years later.* New York: University Press of America.

Perkins-Dock, R. E. (2005). The application of Adlerian family therapy with African American families. *The Journal of Individual Psychology, 61,* 233–249.

Silk, H. J. (2008). A cultural home visit training experience in medical school. *Home Healthcare Management & Practice, 20*(4), 323–327.

Turner, C. W. (2008). *My seven-day makeover: One breast cancer survivor's spiritual journey.* Champaign, IL: 4044 Publishing.

Villarosa, L. (1994). *Body and soul: The Black woman's guide to physical health and emotional well-being.* New York: Harper Collins.

CHAPTER 6

A Granddaughter's Story

Monica R. Robinson

When my grandmother was diagnosed with cancer, the doctors gave us a timeline of six months from that date that my grandmother would probably be alive. It was traumatic for our family—we could not fathom her not being with us. When I first heard that, when they said she wasn't going to make it, I thought: my daughter is going to graduate; I can't imagine my grandmother not seeing my daughter graduate from college, or get married. All these things start running through your mind. My grandmother said that she, in fact, wanted to live. She wanted to fight if there was something she could do to remain here.

As a family, we pulled together and started asking questions: What about this? What about this? What about that? We started doing our own research. The beautiful part of it is that my mom has two brothers and two sisters and they trade off in taking my grandmother for blood work and treatment. It's just so neat—the doctors say my grandmother is a phenomenon because she hasn't gotten sick through the chemo treatment; she hasn't lost her hair. She is a lot more tired after the therapy, but she usually has lunch with whomever takes her to her therapy—which is a good thing. She is able to eat.

She was losing weight—you knew there was something wrong. I would ask her, "Nana, are you okay, is everything okay?" "Oh, yeah, baby, I'm fine. I feel good. Grandma's just a little tired." But I asked, "If you were in pain, would you tell me?" She would just laugh. Now, I really appreciate the fact that she goes to her treatments; she does what she has to do.

The doctor is really good and is appreciative that we came together as a family. We have all these questions—maybe I have a different question, maybe someone else has a different question, so we all come together—sister, daughter, and granddaughter. We just don't *take* what is said. We ask, "Well, what about this?" For instance, we asked about homeopathic products, which he said he would not recommend—but the choice would basically be up to her.

I think the beauty of it has been that we're all here—my mom and her brothers and sisters are here. My grandmother loves to be on time. So if one knows that they have to take her to an appointment, they know they need to be there and be there on time. Even though I don't think it's a big deal if you're a little late, she likes to be on time. The brothers and sisters sit down and talk about the treatment and what my grandmother wants to do. They go to the doctor with her, get information, and ask questions. Overall, I think that support is so important.

Our family support extends to the community. We have a scholarship fund in honor of my grandmother—the Alice V. Haynes Scholarship Award. Every year, my mom and her siblings do that for African American studies. The student recipient can use the scholarship for college tuition or other expenses.

We are family-oriented people. Yes, everybody has his or her own life and does different things, but still, an outpouring of people came to see my grandmother, to spend time with her, to be there with her for whatever it was she needed—so much love and support. We are going to do what we need to do to get through it, to get over the next hump. We are supporting as a family, as an entity, as a whole, as a structure.

I don't have cancer, but I know it could happen at some point in my life. If it does, I hope to have the same support I've been able to give my grandmother. Both sides of our family are very connected. If one of us has cancer, we all basically embrace it. You just jump on board, dig in, and do—pull up your bootstraps, and do whatever you need to do. For instance:

1. Do your own research—know what is going on.
2. We throw out a lot of "what ifs." If this doesn't work, then what? If that doesn't work, then what?" Everybody has different ideas and different thoughts to add to the process.
3. Don't feel as though you can't do something—bring over a meal, something as simple as that. Offer to take your loved one to a treatment—something supportive. Sit down and find out what needs to be done—how can you help? It might be going over and sitting

together. It might be a "girls' day"—go to the movie, out to dinner, or out to lunch.

4. Sometimes you have to say, "I am going to do this" rather than asking "What can I do? How can I help?" You may have to take it upon yourself to say, "Okay, this is what I can do—I will take Dad to his appointment" because family members can become so overwhelmed they just go in circles.

5. If family becomes overwhelmed, or if one of you sees the other getting overwhelmed, then have a family meeting: "This is what I am going to do—this is what you have scheduled to do. Anybody want to change anything?" And go from there.

I know that our support—the fact that the family supports and embraces my grandmother—has gotten her where she needs to be. Once when we took her to therapy, a man asked, "You all sisters?" We went down the chain and told him who everybody was. "Whatever it is, I know you are going to get through it," he said, "because you've got a bunch of beautiful love and support here."

I think as African Americans, we sometimes don't take advantage of a lot of the information that's out there. You have people who, because of their situation or where they are in life, feel it's not proper to ask certain things or to be involved in their family member's medical history. We can create a lot of barriers. Yet, as mentioned earlier, my grandmother's doctor told us that he wanted to commend us on coming in and asking questions. We always tell him we're not trying to be rude or trying to sidestep—we want her here in treatment, so we are trying to find out what can we do. We ask: What about this? What about that? That is just part of medicine; that is just part of what we have to do in this day and age.

Of course, we're all spiritual, so we always say, "I'm praying for you. Our prayers are going up; blessings are coming down. We know that God is good—you are doing what you need to be doing."

Coping in an American Indian Family

CHAPTER 7

Why Me? Why Anybody?

Sharon R. Johnson

A merican Indian families are like any other family—
composed of some wonderful people, and some not so
wonderful. Because of the innate tribal grouping structure, however, the concept of extended family is very
strong in American Indians. In general, readers might
think that any discussion of Indian customs and values applies to all
American Indians, but "there are over 560 federally recognized tribes
and over 100 state recognized tribes, of which each has its own unique
culture" (Intercultural Cancer Council, p. 1).

One of the most terrifying and dreaded moments in a person's life is
that moment when your doctor tells you that you have cancer. After the
initial shock and emotional reaction, your mind floods with questions.
Here are some of the questions you will have at the time of diagnosis,
and for which you and your family will want answers.

1. Why me?

Why you? Maybe it's because you smoked heavily for 30 years. But
maybe you lived a very healthy life and you still have cancer. I don't
know that "Why me?" can be answered. Maybe there is an answer, and
maybe there isn't, but it doesn't matter at this point—*it just doesn't matter.*
Right now, what *does* matter is that you have cancer, and you need to
decide what to do.

2. How bad is this? Will I die? Can this be treated?

Though direct, these are questions that you have to ask. You must find the courage to demand true answers from your doctor. Having someone with you can be of great help—someone who provides both emotional support and another pair of ears, so that later, when you are trying to recall just what was said, there is someone to help you remember.

3. Who will help me?

Initially, you will think about who in your family will help you—your daughter, your husband or partner, your sister, your mother. But there might also be others who can help. For younger adults, there might be a great deal of immediate or extended family—daughters and sons, nieces and nephews, uncles, aunts, and cousins. For older adults, there may not be as many family members available—support systems can dwindle with age (see chapter 2). You might have to search outside your family for someone who can help you, but this could result in a wider range of helpers. For instance, reservation-based Community Health Representatives (http://www.ihs.gov/NonMedicalPrograms/chr/) are trained to provide the type of help that you will need. You may be able to find help through a patient navigator, a person trained to help you make your way through a huge amount of cancer-related information, as well as appointments, treatment choices, and decisions you must make (see chapter 12).

The most important thing? Don't isolate yourself! Don't refuse the help available to you, and do use all resources available. Start with a hospital or clinic social worker, whom your doctor can recommend, and contact the Social Services office at your reservation even if you do not live on the rez. Find out what is available and ask for assistance.

4. How can I tell my family?

Your family has a right to know what is going on—the most difficult thing for people is to not know. Give as much information as you can, try to be calm and comforting, and answer their questions honestly. However, you may at some point have to remind some family members that this is about you, not them, and that you need their support and love.

You will find it much more beneficial to avoid negative people who wail and flail and expect you to give them all your attention. Try not to listen to people who preach doom and gloom. Stay near people who are comforting, helpful, kind, supportive, and caring. We hope this book provides information families and survivors will need, as well as links to Web sites that provide basic, understandable ideas in addition to more complete and scientific information.

5. Who will take care of my family?

This might be a tremendous concern if you are caring for young children. The answer to this question will be different for everyone. Even with an older adult, where immediate child or family member care might not be a concern, there might be questions, such as who will host Thanksgiving dinner.

Your mind will be racing after the diagnosis, and suddenly everything will seem equally important. You will be "whelmed" and then overwhelmed, so remember to slow down and

* Start making lists.
* Start writing down questions that arise.
* Figure out who can help you.
* Start a list of people to call, including phone numbers.

Such preparation serves two purposes: It helps you plan what must happen right away in order to take care of what is most important, and it helps to keep you from useless worry and fear.

6. When can treatment start? How long will this take?

It will seem that your treatment will take longer than you ever thought. It may even take a long time to determine your treatment. Cancer is a chronic disease, and it may result in some form of permanent disability. Your life will be different now.

While in treatment, you will find that cancer will rule your life and that everything you need to do will be planned around your cancer. It may rule your family's life as well. And yet there is no way to hurry the process—everything has to happen in its own good time. The good side of this is that the only thing you have to focus on is today.

You can't make time go by faster or slower, so don't worry about the future. Just take it a day at a time. Enjoy what you can—don't waste precious time just waiting and worrying. There are other things going on around you all the time—people who need your help and support, your care, your love. Focus on that as much as possible.

7. Will I be disfigured? Will I lose my hair?

Possibly. It will depend on what kind of cancer you have. But again, right now that is the least of your problems. That is something to consider and learn about later. And remember this: The people who love you won't care.

8. I am so frightened. I don't want to tell anyone because they will ask questions, and it is too real when I talk about my diagnosis. People will look at me funny and not want to be around me. How can I handle this better?

You have a right to personal privacy, but don't let your own need to be private deprive you from the help and solace of people who are ready to listen and help. If you feel people are looking at you funny, maybe it is because they don't want to offend you, and they just don't know how to offer help.

How can you handle it better? Try not to be frightened—you can cry next week, but right now you are busy. You have to reach out for information and support from both friends and family. Being frightened and crawling into yourself is a luxury you can't afford at the moment. Remember, however, that you don't have to tell everyone everything—you have a right to your privacy. Just don't give up warmth and support from the people around you.

9. Where will the money for treatment come from?

Hopefully you have health insurance, but if you don't have insurance, treatment may be covered through Medicaid, your state's medical assistance program (see chapter 12). Talk with the hospital social worker for advice. Call the Social Security Administration to determine if you are eligible for disability payments. Check with county medical assistance. You will feel a loss of privacy because everyone will want details of your illness, your diagnosis, and your treatment, as well as an income statement from you.

Possibly the Indian Health Service or your tribe can assist you. Call your reservation health provider. If you are not eligible for assistance, you can start looking for other sources. Get all the information you possibly can so you will know what needs to be done next and who can help. It is certainly helpful to have someone help you with paying the bills that need to be paid!

10. Can I trust my doctor? Should I get a second opinion?

Definitely get a second opinion. Even if you trust your doctor, get a second opinion. But remember, a second opinion is usually about determining your best course of treatment, not about whether you have cancer. Because medical tests today are so much better than in the past, most likely you can trust that the doctor has given you the proper diagnosis. Before he or she sits down to talk to you about this, the doctor will have put together all of your test results, and will probably have consulted other doctors about what is wrong and how to treat the problem. But do get a second opinion, if for no other reason than to help you be sure you know about all possible treatments, and that you are choosing the right treatment and have made the right choices.

11. Who has control here? Can I disagree or must I just accept what happens (or what I'm told will happen)?

You have control, and you should insist on keeping that control. No one can treat you without your consent. Regarding your cancer, no one can force you into action that you don't want. If you should decide, for whatever reason, that you do not want to be treated, then that is your right. It is your body, your life, and your choice to make. If you choose to be treated, you have the right to choose what treatment you will receive. If you feel that you are not being allowed to do things the way you want, find someone who will be with you and help you stand up to the people who are trying to make your decisions for you.

12. The hospital wants me to sign papers about something called a *living will*. If I sign a living will, does it mean they will just let me die instead of getting treatment?

No. A living will means that you get to decide what treatment you have. If you want the hospital to do every possible thing to keep you alive, they will. If you say that you don't want to be hooked up to machines for months, no one can make that happen. A living will gives you the power and the right to make your own choices.

13. I don't understand all of these technical terms, but no one will explain this to me in a way that I can understand. What can I do? Where can I get help?

What you can do is speak up. If the doctor keeps going, then say that you need to talk to someone who can tell you in practical, understandable words what is going on. If you reach a point where the technical terms are overwhelming and you are afraid there is no other doctor you can communicate with, find a chaplain, an advocate, or a nurse. Doctors are starting to understand that people want truthful, down-to-earth information, but doctors can be busy. Your doctor is human, but, again, you are in control. It might not be easy, but if you can't speak up to your doctor, take someone with you. Take a teenager. They are good at speaking up!

Don't be afraid to ask for help. Help can even come from a child or grandchild, especially if help is needed using the Internet (see chapter 11). Help with the Internet also could come from a friend, a neighbor, or even from a stranger you meet at the library. Web sites devoted to cancer and American Indians include

* Native C.I.R.C.L.E., The American Indian/Alaska Native Cancer Information Resource Center and Learning Exchange: http://cancercenter.mayo.edu/native.cfm
* Native American Cancer Research: http://natamcancer.org/

14. What do I do about all this paperwork?

Having cancer includes an incredible amount of paperwork. You will sign your name 2,000 times! You will say. "Yes, you told me" and "Yes, I understand." The thing you have to remember is that you can't ignore the paperwork. You have to do it, but you don't have to do it by yourself. There are people in your life who want to help you and who can sort through envelopes and determine what is necessary to deal with and when the paperwork is due. Friends and family can help you make a calendar, fill out papers, or collect information.

Again, lean on children and grandchildren. They are quick and knowledgeable. They can understand things quickly that you might not be able or willing to spend the time to understand. Perhaps because of treatment effects, you can't focus on the paperwork. But don't ignore the paperwork. Find someone to help you.

15. I don't understand about insurance, and they are asking me to send information. Who can help me with this?

If you have insurance, you should have an insurance agent. Call your agent and ask for help. Again, get your paperwork team to help you. They can at least read through the paperwork and ask if you have the information requested, if you want to give the information, or if you know where to get the information.

Again, don't ignore it. If your insurance carrier has agreed to pay for something, you may be asked to sign one more sheet of paper before they mail the check. Find someone who can help you keep track and get things filled out and mailed.

16. What about my job? Can I work?

Your insurance may be tied to your job, so you will be concerned about keeping your job if you have one. Sit down with someone who can help you look at your priorities—for instance, keeping your insurance and having access to treatment.

You might experience fatigue or loss of functioning of part of the body, leading to temporary or permanent disability. The Americans with Disabilities Act (also known as ADA) prohibits some types of job discrimination against people who have or have had cancer by employers (who have at least 15 employees), employment agencies, and labor unions (see chapter 12). Additionally, every state has a law that regulates, to some extent, disability-based employment discrimination. It is important for you to understand disability-related concepts such as *reasonable accommodation*, which means that an employer can support you by altering your work or work schedule in some way to accommodate, for instance, fatigue due to chemotherapy.

If you don't have a job, but want one, cancer or its treatment may result in a disability. For individuals experiencing a disability that impacts employment, vocational rehabilitation (VR) can offer a solution (http://www.ed.gov/programs/rsabvrs/index.html). Public VR services have been integrated into U.S. legislation since 1917. The public VR system, which is both state and federal in terms of funding and regulations, is rooted in the 1935 Social Security Act and is strengthened by the Rehabilitation Act of 1973 and its subsequent amendments. Public VR is provided by state agencies, but primarily funded and regulated by a federal agency, the Rehabilitation Services Administration (RSA). Each state has its own department of vocational rehabilitation.

There is also private for-profit VR as well as tribal VR. An important resource for tribal VR is the Consortia of Administrators for Native American Rehabilitation (CANAR; see http://www.canar.org). The mission of CANAR is to facilitate collaboration and cooperation among administrators of rehabilitation projects serving Native American persons with disabilities, resulting in positive outcomes for Native American persons with disabilities. Individual tribal VR programs are listed at http://www.canar.org/map.php, but if your tribe doesn't have a tribal VR program, you can always be served by the public VR program.

VR programs help individuals with physical or mental disabilities to obtain employment and live more independently through the provision of such supports as counseling, medical and psychological services, job training, and other individualized services.

A plan for rehabilitation services is obtained through a counseling and/or assessment process that engages applicants and clients fully in actively exploring their vocational interests, abilities, capabilities, and service/process options, as well as in making choices. RSA's funds to state VR agencies require that priority be given to providing services to individuals who are deemed significantly disabled; the VR program is considered to be an eligibility program and not an entitlement program. The preferred goal of VR services is economic independence (i.e., full-time employment); however, other outcomes are possible, such as independent living (versus some sort of group or shelter-type facility), self-employment, and even what is referred to as homemaker services or unpaid family worker.

Two resources that can help you begin to understand cancer as a disability and its impact on work include

* *Cancer and the Workplace Part I: The Challenge of Creating Supportive Work Environments for Employees with Cancer and their Caregivers*. Listen to this archived Telephone Education Workshop, a free educational seminar available for people with cancer, their loved ones and health-care professionals: http://www.cancercare.org/get_help/tew_archive/practical_concerns.php
* *Working It Out: Your Employment Rights As A Cancer Survivor*. Barbara Hoffman, JD, Founding Chair, National Coalition for Cancer Survivorship (NCCS): http://www.canceradvocacy.org/resources/publications/employment.pdf

Reference

Intercultural Cancer Council. *American Indians/Alaska Natives & Cancer*. Retrieved November 6, 2009, from http://iccnetwork.org/cancerfacts/ICC-CFS2.pdf, p. 1).

Coping in an Asian American Family

CHAPTER 8

Trees Don't Mourn the Autumn: A Creative Response

Alice F. Chang, with Paul Donnelly

> Happy families are all alike; every unhappy family is unhappy in its own way.
>
> *Anna Karenina*, Leo Tolstoy

Cancer can enter a family like a meteor, suddenly and with burning force. Or it can enter a family like a pebble dropped into a still pond, gaining force as the ripples travel from the point of impact. Either way, it is always a shock to everyone involved, whether consciously acknowledged or not.

Anticipated or unanticipated, there is an absolute line of demarcation between the time before a diagnosis and the time after. A family's strengths and weaknesses may become highlighted. The dynamics of a family may change in unexpected ways. Understanding and coping with these changes contributes to the heart and soul of healing.

There is clearly no one model for a family's response to a cancer diagnosis, nor one model for the "typical Asian family." Filipino? South Asian? Japanese? Korean? Vietnamese? Chinese? Hmong? Tolstoy's great observation certainly applies to families struggling with cancer in their midst: "Every unhappy family is unhappy in its own way."

This is not to say that culture isn't significant or that European models should be primary. Culture forms a vivid and distinctive part of our experience and of our voices as cancer patients and as the families of people with cancer. Respect for elders, stoicism, and reticence are not necessarily constraining, just as volubility, praying the rosary aloud, or emotional gatherings are not necessarily excesses. When families are touched by cancer, the way in which they respond publicly and the way in which they respond in private may not be the same. Culture often plays a vital role in a family's response. Culture can define the degree to which family members may acknowledge that a disease even exists in the family.

When a seemingly private affair becomes too public, it may bring dismay to some and joy to others. Family members often give subtle cues and "cries for help" that may be misread by both the family and their community. For instance, members of Asian American families and communities may feel compelled to observe an especially strong distinction between what may be acknowledged publicly and what may only be acknowledged privately—what is acknowledged privately may have meaning only to oneself.

Case Example 1: A Chinese American Family

Consider the case of a 45-year-old Chinese American woman who complained to her primary care physician of pain in her stomach region. Her blood work showed that she was a little anemic, so the physician told her to take iron pills and eat more protein because she was slight in build. She refused to tell anyone how badly she felt, not even her husband, because she didn't want to upset anyone in the family.

After nearly three years, her physician told her that her continued pain must be the result of a "nervous stomach from job stress." He prescribed a tranquilizer and antacids. A knowledgeable family member noted that this didn't make much sense, because she was generally healthy and certainly not a person prone to anxiety. The relative encouraged her to seek further diagnostic tests, but since she could still stand the pain in her lower back and abdomen, she thought further testing was unnecessary.

Eventually, however, the pain was so horrific that she wasn't able to eat and thus lost 20–30 pounds. The relative remembered that the woman's father had died two weeks after suddenly informing her (his only child) that he had stomach cancer. The father had not said anything to the woman because he didn't want to upset her, not realizing that, as a result, she and his grandchildren were given no time to prepare and were unable to help him for the nine months during which he knew he was dying. The sudden and powerful loss of his death had left the woman feeling depressed, helpless, hopeless, and angry that her father had not shared his final illness.

The relative reminded the woman that she had been an adult—40 years old—when she heard from her father that he had cancer, and asked if she wanted her children, who were teenagers, to face a similar situation on such short notice should she too have stomach cancer. The relative told her not to be "Chinese Proud," but rather to go and sit at the doctor's office until they found out what was really wrong with her body (notice, not what was wrong with *her*, but what was wrong with her body). Fortunately, the woman and her husband gave that advice some thought and returned to the doctor's office for further tests.

The test results showed that the woman had advanced pancreatic cancer and had a short time to live. Her children were informed immediately. The relative who was more familiar with cancer care insisted that she be treated, at least for palliative care. When in less pain, the woman rallied for a bit and was even able to eat. Family members had an opportunity to enjoy moments together that they would have missed if she had remained silent prior to a sudden death—keeping her illness private and known only to herself. They were able to plan together the ritual she preferred for her memorial service. The woman died 18 months later, and the family was thankful to have had the opportunity to prepare with her. It did not lessen the pain and sorrow of the loss, but it helped.

While this woman and mother ultimately served as a role model of the values of hope and resilience, and the time the family had together contributed to the emotional resources that they developed to cope with their feelings of grief and loss, a period of warning before death can be a double-edged sword. This time can help families prepare for the loss of a loved one, but it also can be a time of foreboding, even a time during which the family feels disgraced. The time following diagnosis contains a yin and a yang of cohesion and crisis, of threat and opportunity.

Case Example 2: A Filipino American Family

In speaking of her mother's stomach cancer, a Filipina community leader described her family's devastation at discovering that her mother had been misdiagnosed several times and had spent two years taking ever-larger doses of antacids. When her mother was finally taken to the emergency room for weakness and bleeding, tests found so much fluid in her stomach that she had to have a catheter installed for drainage. An advanced tumor was discovered shortly thereafter. As her illness progressed, the family veered between devastation and stoicism. Her surgeon was brusque and pessimistic, while her oncologist was more gentle and encouraging. Suffice it to say that she survived the surgeon's prognosis by more than a year.

The last time she was in the hospital, the family thought she would bounce back as always. Her three children made sure she had visitors in addition to their father. Seeing her grandchildren brought her joy and lifted her spirits. Everyone in the family, immediate and extended, brought things they thought she would want to eat.

As she weakened and began to have bouts of disorientation, calls went out to the rest of the family. She was the matriarch of a large extended family. She, a younger brother, and a younger sister were the last survivors among eight siblings. Her last days became a communal experience, with extended family staying in the room and many others passing in and out. In the way of Filipino Catholics, the group spent its time reminiscing and praying. Some older members of the family and community wept and keened in anticipatory grief. It was, all in all, a vibrant and tumultuous scene and not at all in the typical European model of still figures and hushed voices

As her end became imminent, the immediate family was left to have a final farewell. The dying woman's husband would not leave the room, telling his three children, "just bring me things." And they did as they were told, as this was a time to offer respect, not advice.

Although this Filipino family had an extensive and effective support network, the lack of formal resources in the community also became apparent. There seemed to be no support groups—not for patients, not for families, and not for the bereaved—that understood Filipino cultural needs or were language specific. "Well, they were very language specific: English." This community leader is determined to make some sense of her experience and offer tribute to her mother by advocating for the establishment of culturally and linguistically appropriate support groups for Filipino cancer patients, their families, and the bereaved in Southern California.

However, creating community resources for use by Asian Americans can be impeded by the Asian American cultural bent to be strong, to be stoic, to be private, and to endure. Cultural values include not acknowledging weakness, which often can mean physical or mental illness, as well as inabilities to cope with such illnesses.

Giving Back

The outcome of being touched by cancer often causes champions or survivors to contribute newly gained energy and knowledge to future cancer patients and their families, as well as to the community at large. For instance, as a survivor of breast cancer, I (Alice F. Chang) have made an effort to give back to my community by founding in 1995, along with John J. Welker and his wife, the late Gertrude Welker, The Academy for Cancer Wellness (ACW), a 501 (c)(3) nonprofit organization. Its purpose is to provide support for cancer wellness—for champions, as well as for their families and friends. Our mission:

> To spread awareness of the many people who have faced the challenge of cancer and emerged triumphant; to provide a means for cancer champions to rally amongst themselves for mutual strength and support; to provide funding for research toward the promotion of cancer wellness; and to provide modest financial support for the working poor and under-insured cancer patients. (www.cancerhealth.org)

A number of benefit concerts have provided support for our work honoring cancer champions and supporting treatment for cancer patients in need. ACW allows me to use the time I have been given to do good. I have also tried to make sense of my experience by telling my story in ways that may be helpful to others. My book, *A Survivor's Guide to Breast Cancer,* combines frank reflections on my own illness and course of treatment with facts about treatment and concrete suggestions for coping with each aspect of diagnosis, treatment, and recovery.

I might never have thought to turn aspects of my story into a play had I not known Paul Donnelly. The short version: We were already acquainted when he was asked to interview me for a newsletter article. The more of my story he heard, the more interested he became. He told me that I had given him much too much material for a newsletter article. We took a few months to get to know one another better and then embarked on the project that became a play, *Trees Don't Mourn the Autumn.* Here, we share four scenes from the much longer work. The main character, Emily Lin, is a psychologist and a breast cancer survivor. Emily's diagnosis, treatment, and recovery form the through line of the play, with digressions to her nightmares, her early life, her disastrous first marriage, and her reunion with a child she had long ago given up for adoption.

The title of the play is drawn from "Within Measured Boundaries," an article by Jenilu Schoolman, a psychologist who wrote movingly about her own 11-year battle with breast cancer:

"In this crisis, I watch the cycle of the seasons. Trees do not mourn their autumn as the leaves fall at the appointed time. New ones are ready to replace them" (http://oreilly.com/medical/breastcancer/news/faith.html).

In the numberless ways that a cancer diagnosis can be a shock to family members, it is clearly also a shock to the cancer patient. The following scene from *Trees Don't Mourn the Autumn* captures the moment when awareness of the truth of her illness dawns upon Emily, and the coin fully drops. I hope Emily's story—my story—and the struggle to understand and accept a cancer diagnosis will resonate for many family members.

Setting: Dr. Hudson's Office, January 1994.

DR. HUDSON   Emily . . . Emily . . . Are you all right?

EMILY (from behind the screen)   I'll just be a little bit longer.

DR. HUDSON   I'm sorry. I know that's a particularly stupid question . . .
 under the circumstances.

 EMILY bursts from behind the screen. She is in street clothes that have clearly been donned in haste. She is still pulling on a shoe as she appears.

EMILY Sorry . . . sorry, didn't mean to hold you up.

DR. HUDSON No, *I'm* sorry. I didn't mean to rush you. (holding out a chair) Here. Sit for a minute. Catch your breath.

EMILY I'm sorry. This has all been so sudden. A week ago I was a healthy person with a muscle pull . . . and now . . . it's just all so sudden. Not that I don't appreciate you seeing me so quickly. I do. I appreciate it very much. I was so surprised when your office called at 2 to say you had a cancellation at 4. I was very grateful. When I first called, the young lady told me you didn't have an opening for three weeks. I was glad not to have to wait. But then I had this terrible panic when I stopped by the radiologist's to pick up the x-rays. There wouldn't be all this rush if something wasn't terribly wrong. But then I told myself that couldn't be right . . . it's been so painful, it couldn't be serious . . . it couldn't be . . . well, you know. Is it? Is it . . . how bad is it?

DR. HUDSON Well, Emily, I don't think we need to panic. I'll certainly try to pull my foot back off the accelerator a little and give you some time to absorb things.

EMILY What things?

DR. HUDSON. You haven't seen the x-rays yet, have you?

EMILY No.

DR. HUDSON Let's have a look together.

EMILY All right.

DR. HUDSON Here. This is your right breast. (slide shows x-ray) You can see how clear and relatively even . . .

EMILY Yes, yes . . . and the other?

DR. HUDSON I think you can see the differences.

EMILY nods.

DR. HUDSON Where it is darker . . . from here to here . . . that indicates some kind of an abnormality. And these little bursts of light . . .

EMILY Star asterisk clusters.

DR. HUDSON Yes. Do you know what they usually indicate?

EMILY Sites of calcification, right?

DR. HUDSON Yes. But, I'm afraid these are almost always indicative of a malignancy.

EMILY stiffens.

DR. HUDSON I'm sorry. In 20 years I haven't found the right way to tell someone she has cancer.

EMILY Why are you telling me?

DR. HUDSON We need a biopsy, of course, to confirm . . . but I'm afraid the indications are pretty clear.

EMILY I hear you and I guess what you are saying is true. I've worked with so many women . . . and yet, now, I can't believe . . . it just doesn't feel like we're talking about me. I've seen x-rays like this before . . . and

I feel for that woman and I hope I can help her . . . but I can't possibly be her!

DR. HUDSON   I know it's not easy. And you don't need to make any decisions today. In fact, I won't let you. But we need to talk about options. If you need to come back and hear them again, we can talk again. But we have to start a conversation today.

EMILY nods.

DR. HUDSON   This part *has* gotten easier over the past 20 years, Emily. A lot easier. I have better . . . less intrusive, less debilitating options to offer . . . and when we get to treatments, there's real hope today. It's not going to be an easy path, but it is one that is likely to lead to recovery. And that wasn't often the case when I was starting out. I know that's not much comfort right this minute . . .

EMILY   No. 'Fibrous mass.' 'Cyst.' 'Fibroid.' Hearing them would be a comfort.

DR. HUDSON   Yes. And hearing otherwise is an awful shock. One that you can't prepare for no matter what you might have suspected or feared . . .

EMILY   I never considered . . . and I'm not convinced. That technician wasn't very good, you know. She kept squeezing and adjusting . . . Someone who knew her business wouldn't have needed that many exposures . . .

DR. HUDSON   We need a biopsy to be certain of anything, but, in the meantime, may I sketch out a hypothetical course of treatment . . . a 'just in case' scenario.

EMILY   I don't know. My life is already in an uproar. I'm just starting to get my practice going here. Right now I'm barely making my basic living expenses. I can't be sick now. I can't . . . If I can't work, I have no income. If I have no income, I can't pay my deductible . . . never mind my mortgage. This hypothetical conversation sounds like an unnecessary stressor to me!

DR. HUDSON   I'd like to hope it will be just the opposite . . . That it may ground us and help alleviate some of your anxiety.

EMILY   Somehow I doubt it. But go ahead.

DR. HUDSON   We'll start with the biopsy. As you probably know, all biopsy procedures remove a tissue sample for microscopic evaluation. We have two primary options. The fine-needle biopsy can be done here in the office. As the name suggests, I will insert a thin needle into the breast and withdraw some tissue. If we find we need a larger sample, then I'd perform an excisional biopsy. That would be done on an outpatient basis, most likely under a local anesthesia. I'd make an incision and remove a larger sample.

EMILY   You know that every procedure has to be pre-certified by my insurance company . . . I can't agree to anything without their approval.

DR. HUDSON   Lauren has her whip and chair at the ready . . .

EMILY   I beg your pardon?

DR. HUDSON I'm sorry . . . my office manager has yet to encounter an insurance company she can't tame.

EMILY (smiling) That will be a big help.

DR. HUDSON She's wonderful. And we find doing what we can to lighten that load makes a huge difference for our patients. In either case, we'll have time to discuss treatment options with your full team after we have results . . .

EMILY My "team"?

DR. HUDSON At the minimum, we'll have a radiologist and an oncologist working with us . . .

EMILY Only if it's not a fibroid . . .

DR. HUDSON I'd like to go ahead and help you make some appointments, if you don't mind . . .

EMILY I don't know . . .

DR. HUDSON How would you counsel a patient?

EMILY To trust her instincts . . . to retain her autonomy . . .

DR. HUDSON We're of one mind there. What are your instincts really telling you?

EMILY doesn't answer.

DR. HUDSON Emily?

EMILY To run like hell.

DR. HUDSON I'll bet they are. And I don't blame you for feeling that way. But I really hope you'll trust me a little bit further . . .

EMILY (not convinced) Go on.

DR. HUDSON Being relatively new in town, I assume you haven't had an opportunity to get to know the medical community . . .

EMILY No.

DR. HUDSON Not that many lifelong residents keep a radiologist or an oncologist on call. I can think of several good people in both areas if you want to look at a variety of options or want to ask around. Although, for my money, I don't think you'll beat Billy Siwek and Peter Alpert.

EMILY I could start with them, I suppose . . .

DR. HUDSON I'll have Lauren call for you now, so you can be all set before you leave here today . . .

EMILY Hold on. I have to be in Washington for a meeting on Friday . . .

DR. HUDSON This is only Tuesday. I'm sure Billy and Peter will do their best to see you before you have to leave, or, at worst, as soon as you get back. When will that be?

EMILY Sunday. I leave Thursday afternoon.

DR. HUDSON I'll get Lauren right on it and then come back so we can talk some more . . .

EMILY Oh my . . .

DR. HUDSON   Is that all right?

EMILY   I don't like this sense of urgency. I don't like it one bit.

DR. HUDSON   Think of it as "better safe than sorry."

EMILY   I'm already feeling sorry.

DR. HUDSON (taking EMILY's hand)   I will do everything in my power to make sure that you will never be sorry for trusting me. Okay?

EMILY   I guess I have to be, for now.

DR. HUDSON   I'll always take "for now." I'll be right back.

   DR. HUDSON exits.

Considering Culture in Family Response to Cancer

Case Example 3: A Japanese American Family

A Japanese American's experience with his mother's cancer illustrates the way culture can shape both filial and marital responses to serious illness. This professional, well-educated man's mother experienced three bouts of cancer in 15 years: cervical, for which she had a hysterectomy; breast, for which she had a mastectomy; and cancer of the esophagus. His father had been well enough to take his wife to and from treatment for cervical cancer. Now, the father's Alzheimer's diagnosis and bouts of dementia required that the son, his three brothers, and their spouses take full responsibility for providing any assistance she might need—which they did willingly. Despite their diligent research, the causes and courses of each of their mother's cancers were different—the four "boys" felt guilty for being perpetually behind the necessary learning curve in understanding each different cancer.

Yet the brothers were inspired by their mother's will to live throughout her cancer experiences, by her positive attitude, and by traditional Japanese stoicism. The father's "typically Japanese cultural style"—unsympathetic, expecting his wife to be a servant to the male of the household—was exacerbated by his bouts of dementia. He would scold and become belligerent, she would become withdrawn, and the four siblings would try to keep matters from escalating.

That cancer does not occur in a vacuum is among the most difficult and frustrating aspects of being a cancer patient or caregiver. Other life issues do not recede. The struggle to find balance and to give and accept permission to handle things less than perfectly offers one more unwelcome challenge.

A saving grace of this family's experience with esophageal cancer was finding a culturally appropriate oncologist, a Japanese American from Hawaii who was able to support the brothers. As is the way of life, one load is lifted so another may be borne. As their father's Alzheimer's symptoms worsened, the brothers got him a caretaker during the day and took turns providing evening care for their parents. Their mother was too weak to withstand her final bouts of radiation and died from complications last year at the age of 91.

In *Trees Don't Mourn the Autumn,* Emily imagines how her aging parents, Walter and Agnes, will respond to a call telling them that she may have breast cancer. As proud immigrants, their values and behaviors are rooted in those of their home country. As with much of the creative enterprise, this scene is in some part truth and in some part invention, and explains that for some families, a traditional cultural response may seem insensitive and unfeeling, yet can be understood as the way an older generation was brought up to respond. In fact, the western societal expectation of how things "should" be, of how family members "should" respond, can make the cancer experience more difficult for a cancer patient and his or her family.

Setting: WALTER is seated at a table working with bark and sphagnum moss to prepare community pots for replanting orchid seedlings. AGNES stands behind him.

WALTER   Who was that?

AGNES   Emily.

> WALTER does not respond further.   He has no particular interest in EMILY's life or curiosity about the call.

> AGNES is clearly fretful.

WALTER (finally, with a sigh)   What did she say that gives you need to disrupt my work at this delicate juncture?

AGNES   She has some bad news.

WALTER   We have no money to send her . . .

AGNES   She wasn't asking . . .

WALTER   Not directly, I'm sure. She's the sly one. Too clever to ask directly.

AGNES   She may have cancer.

> WALTER immediately returns to his labors.   He uses tweezers to pick a seedling from a bowl of fungicide solution and place it in the community bowl. He uses the tweezers to position moss loosely over the seedling's roots.

AGNES   Breast cancer. Possibly. She said it wasn't definite. She's having a biopsy next week to confirm.

WALTER   Then why didn't she wait until next week to call?

AGNES   I think she knows already, but she didn't want me to be alarmed.

WALTER   If she didn't want you to be alarmed, why did she call?

AGNES   For comfort.

WALTER   Typical. Concerned only for her own comfort.

   WALTER continues intently with his work.

AGNES   Walter . . .

WALTER   Yes?

AGNES   I . . .

WALTER   Yes?

AGNES   What time will you want to stop for supper?

WALTER   I will be ready in about two hours.

   WALTER continues working. Agnes does not go away.

WALTER   At least we may take some comfort in knowing that this is the last shame *she* will bring upon this family.

Case Example 4: A Vietnamese American Family

To be diagnosed with stomach cancer when your grandson is three months old seems a terrible betrayal. Fortunately for his family, this retired Vietnamese American scientist recently joined in his grandson's 15th birthday celebration. His daughter, an academic (and mother of his grandson), reports that the diagnosis came as a huge shock to the family because her father was "such a health food nut."

Theirs was not a "typical Asian family." Her father was comfortable with doctors and with asking for help. Yet he still found the process difficult due to the inherent lack of control faced by most patients. Despite the family's research and education and resources, "the surgeons did what they do and removed two-thirds of his stomach with no discussion of the impact or of the process of postsurgical recovery."

Both of his daughters and their mother found it difficult to see him appear to age rapidly. Preparing and enjoying food was an important part of the family's time together, and now eating caused him pain, which led to further weight loss. Still, his daughter doesn't feel that culture had a significant impact on this family's experience: "Things weren't withheld; communication channels were open about feelings as well as facts."

In *Trees Don't Mourn the Autumn,* as the date for Emily's surgery approaches, her doctor attempts to establish who might be the members of her support network. Emily Lin finds her voice, knowing that she mustn't let herself be shoehorned into a cultural model that doesn't fit the truth of her experience:

DR. HUDSON   And your family of origin?

EMILY   My parents are both still alive. They're in their eighties. He's a retired academic. They live in Oakland.

DR. HUDSON   And how would you characterize your relationship with them?

EMILY   Correct. I pay them an obligatory visit two or three times a year. I call my mother every week or so just to make sure they're okay.

DR. HUDSON   So they're not going to be much of a source of support?

EMILY   No. I wouldn't dream . . . No. He has a pension and social security. And they have some investments, but they live very hand-to-mouth. It's a reflex among Chinese immigrants of their generation.

DR. HUDSON   I meant emotional support . . .

EMILY laughs quite heartily.

DR. HUDSON   Emily?

EMILY   That would be even less likely.

DR. HUDSON   Why?

EMILY   As I said, they were typical immigrants of their generation.

DR. HUDSON   Meaning . . .

EMILY   They faced a lot of struggle. Everything they were at home was stripped away when they entered an alien and pretty hostile culture. He came for graduate school in the thirties. He was a good student and a good scientist. He was evidently a good teacher of other people's children.

DR. HUDSON   Oh?

EMILY   When colleagues would speak of his kindness or generosity, our family was always sure they had to be talking about someone else.

DR. HUDSON   And the rest of your family?

EMILY   We're not close.

DR. HUDSON   Who's "we"?

EMILY   I have a brother and a sister. I was the youngest. Margaret was the eldest. And Frank was, and is, the prince. Frank wasn't raised to care for anyone other than himself.

DR. HUDSON   It sounds like it was difficult for you.

EMILY   I was unplanned and distinctly unwanted. They were already "burdened" with one daughter. The birth of a second daughter was the tragedy that blighted their lives.

DR. HUDSON   And this was made clear to you?

EMILY   "Every day, in every way . . ." They actually gave me away, for a while, to a childless couple they knew.

DR. HUDSON   No!

EMILY   Oh, yes. I have no memory, of course. I was only a few weeks old. When I'd been with them almost a year, the couple, they became pregnant. If they had had a boy, I would have stayed with them and been a resident handmaiden. Much to the dismay of all, they too were "cursed" with a daughter, and they shamed my parents into taking me back when I was about 22 months old.

DR. HUDSON   That's extraordinary.

EMILY   It set the pattern. When Margaret started junior high school, they decided she was old enough to take care of me. After that they would take Frank on vacations and trips and leave Margaret and me at home.

DR. HUDSON   Are you and Margaret close?

EMILY   Not particularly.

DR. HUDSON   It just seems as though you might have been natural allies . . .

EMILY   It took all the energy and concentration and resources Margaret and I could muster to survive childhood, to get out and to build our separate lives. There wasn't a lot left over for bonding. Sometimes the only life you can afford to save is your own, you know?

DR. HUDSON (shaking her head)   I'd be lying if I said I did. But I believe you. I don't suppose there's any chance . . .

EMILY   Of what?

DR. HUDSON   That your family . . . or even your sister . . . might rise to the occasion? Might what you're going through be extraordinary enough to make a different kind of connection?

EMILY   NO! There's no "Hallmark Halls of Fame" in the offing here, Dr. Hudson! Let me be absolutely clear. There is no place for my parents or my siblings in any of this. They are not to be informed or consulted in any way. Do you understand?

DR. HUDSON   Yes.

EMILY   I put myself through school, doctor. College and grad school. I built a career and an identity and a life alone. Alone. And I will do what has to be done now, alone. Until I just can't do it anymore.. . . And then I'll stop.

Emily doesn't stop. She accepts the support of friends. She is finally able to put the memory of that miserable first marriage behind her. And she reunites with her daughter, Allison, whom she hasn't seen in nearly 30 years. As the play draws to a close, Emily gets a call from her daughter on Super Bowl Sunday, ostensibly to thank her for her Christmas gift. The gift was an antique jade brush and mirror that belonged to Emily's grandmother and that her feckless husband had pawned at the end of their marriage:

Setting: The phone rings. As EMILY goes to answer it, lights come up on ALLISON holding a phone.

ALLISON is nearly six months pregnant and is beginning to show.

EMILY (into the receiver)   Ice.

ALLISON   Excuse me?

EMILY   Oh gosh, Allison! Hello! I'm sorry . . .

ALLISON   That's okay. "Ice"?

EMILY   I'm having a little Super Bowl gathering. I assumed you were someone calling to ask what you could bring.

ALLISON   Well, then, I won't keep you . . .

EMILY   I've got plenty of time. The help just arrived, so everything is under control.

DARRYL (a friend) sticks out his tongue on 'the help,' then exits.

ALLISON   Sounds like fun.

EMILY   It's the first time in a while I've been up to having people in. It should be very nice. What about you? How were your holidays?

ALLISON   Really great. And I really, really want to thank you for your beautiful gift.. . . It really meant . . . (her voice breaks) . . . so much. Shit! I wanted to wait until I could talk about them without crying. Looks like I didn't wait quite long enough.

EMILY   That's okay. I'm so glad you liked them . . .

ALLISON   I did. I do. Very much.

EMILY   I'm glad. I was afraid I might be pushing too hard . . .

ALLISON   Not at all.

EMILY   And I'm sure you've been busy with the holidays. I was afraid they might make things more difficult with your mother.

ALLISON   No. If anything, they seemed to help her understand.

EMILY   Good. That's good.

ALLISON   And I have news that helped. And which may help explain why I have been so emotional lately.

EMILY   What's that?

ALLISON   You sitting down?

EMILY   What? What is it?

ALLISON   I'm going to have a baby.

EMILY is speechless.

ALLISON   Did you hear me?

EMILY nods mutely.

ALLISON   Emily?

EMILY   Oh, Allison . . .

ALLISON   It's supposed to be good news.

EMILY   It is. It's wonderful.

ALLISON   Yes, it is. Michael is so excited I think he's getting even less sleep than me.

EMILY   Tell him not to waste the sleepless nights now. He'll get plenty of them later.. . . Do you . . .

ALLISON   A little girl. Catherine Agnes. You'll have to come visit . . .

EMILY   May I? I would love to. If it won't be a problem . . .

ALLISON She'll take a little more coaxing. But she'll come around.

EMILY Are you sure?

ALLISON No.

EMILY Well . . .

ALLISON But I'm not sure about anything, you know?

EMILY Yes.

ALLISON I'm just beginning to get a clue as to how hard it must have been for you. It's really not possible to imagine, is it?

EMILY No, it's not.

ALLISON Okay. I'm going to let you get back to setting up your party. But I hope you'll come for the christening.

EMILY I wouldn't miss it.

ALLISON Good.

EMILY I'll give you a call real soon.

ALLISON I'd like that. 'Bye for now.

EMILY 'Bye.

  As they each set down their receivers, lights fade out on ALLISON.

DARRYL (returning) I was trying not to get caught listening . . .

  EMILY sits.

DARRYL Em?

DARRYL I take it she liked the mirror and brush?

  EMILY nods.

DARRYL Maybe someday you'll stop worrying about everything.

EMILY You just can't ever know.. . . . You can never predict . . .

DARRYL How could she not appreciate a jade mirror and brush? Never mind the sentimental value, they were beautiful pieces . . .

EMILY No. You can never predict . . .

DARRYL What?

EMILY Where life will take you next . . .

DARRYL What's going on now?

EMILY You can never know how bad it's going to be sometimes. And then you can't guess how wonderful it can be others.

DARRYL If I stop asking will you tell me?

EMILY I like this year's news a whole lot better!

DARRYL And that "news" is?

  EMILY is again speechless.

DARRYL What, already? What?

EMILY A sentence I truly never thought I'd say . . .

DARRYL Oh, boy . . .

EMILY   Close. Oh, girl.

DARRYL   When did you get so didactic? (getting it) Oh, my . . .

EMILY (nodding)   I'm going to be a grandmother. Me.

DARRYL   Congratulations.

   EMILY doesn't respond.

DARRYL   This is a good thing, right?

EMILY   Yes.

DARRYL   Your enthusiasm is breathtaking.

EMILY   When you never held your own child, it doesn't even cross your mind that you might hold a grandchild someday. I'm stunned. But I'm here. Bald and aching, but about to be a grandmother.

   Lights fade to BLACK.

<u>CURTAIN</u>
End of *Trees Don't Mourn the Autumn*

One trait I share with Emily is amazement at how far I have come from where I expected to be at the start of my cancer journey. I did not write much—for one thing, my arm hurt too much—during my recovery. But having written *A Survivor's Guide to Breast Cancer* and co-authored *Trees Don't Mourn the Autumn,* I understand how therapeutic writing can be. I did both in the hope that others would benefit from my experience, and I have found satisfaction in having that hope fulfilled.

Many books and Web sites promote the value of journaling and other forms of creative expression for reducing stress and even promoting healing among cancer patients. Popular Web sites and media also promote journaling and other forms of creative expression for the general public. It seems reasonable to suggest that the family members of cancer patients would also benefit from journaling or, if writing doesn't sound appealing, drawing or painting or playing an instrument or any other form of self-expression. Coping can certainly be enhanced by journaling or dance or painting, but music may offer the fullest model, with the opportunity to simply listen or to play a soothing piece or pound away at drums with energy and volume, with rage or with joy. The most important thing is to find the form or expression that feels most helpful to you.

In this chapter, I have used a series of scenes from my play to show that one generalization about Asian Americans that may have a grain of truth is that we can be reserved, impassive, or fearful of expressing emotion. We might very well benefit from a private outlet for the feelings stirred by having a loved one with cancer. A feeling may be expressed usefully in writing or painting or music or dance without necessarily being shared.

There are some hard-and-fast truths about Asian Americans that may not be well known. Here are just a few of the many disturbing research findings from "The Unequal Burden of Cancer Among Asian Americans," assembled by the Asian American Network for Cancer Awareness, Research and Training (AANCART):

* While heart disease is the leading cause of death for all U.S. groups (all ages), cancer has been the number-one killer of Asian American women since 1980.
* Filipinos have the second poorest five-year survival rates for colon and rectal cancers of all U.S. ethnic groups (second to American Indians).
* Lung cancer rates among Southeast Asians are 18% higher than among white Americans.
* Cervical cancer incidence rates in Vietnamese women are five times higher than the rate among white American women.
* The incidence of liver cancer in Chinese, Filipino, Japanese, Korean, and Vietnamese populations are 1.7 to 11.3 times higher than rates among white Americans.

AANCART is a cooperative agreement between the National Cancer Institute (NCI) and the University of California, Davis. The AANCART Web site (http://www.aancart.org/) has a wealth of information about the incidence of cancer in Asian American communities and educational resources.

Any steps that each of us is able to take, from attention to our own health to public advocacy, will help to address the unequal burden of cancer in our community. By reducing the number of cancer patients, we reduce the number of family members affected by cancer. According to the 2000 U.S. Census, the average size of an Asian American household was 3.51. That's the standard "nuclear" family living under one roof, so when the true family dynamic of adult children, siblings, parents, aunts, uncles, and cousins is factored in, each individual's cancer affects many more than 3.51 family members.

We may not be able to eliminate cancer, but we can reduce its disparate impact on our community and its devastating impact on our families. This writing will be worthwhile if it leads to families who are less unhappy in the short term and fewer unhappy families over time.

Coping in a Latino Family

Listening with the Heart to "Unspoken" Needs: Latina Perspectives on Coping and Living with Cancer

Alma E. Flores, Claudia X. Aguado Loi, Gloria I. San Miguel, and Dinorah (Dina) Martinez Tyson

> Cancer is a very difficult illness, but it unites families. . . . We have families waiting for us, children that need our presence in their lives, parents that miss us, and friends willing to give us all their support. Cancer is a difficult illness, not only for those diagnosed with it, but also for those around us.
>
> Mayte Prida, 2005
> Translated from *Una Etapa Dificil: Mi Lucha Contra EL Cancer*
> *(A Difficult Phase: My Battle Against Cancer)*

We hope that reading this chapter will provide you, the co-survivor, with both the strength and some useful tools to embark on your cancer journey with your loved one without losing your sense of direction. For the professional care provider, we hope to provide easy-to-implement strategies for tuning in to the "unspoken" needs of Latinos touched by cancer. In this chapter, you will find anecdotes and testimonials gathered from *pláticas* (conversations) with survivors and co-survivors, statements from support group meetings, excerpts from our literature review, survey findings, and Camp Alegria evaluations (Martinez, Aguado Loi, Martinez, Flores, & Meade, 2008), all interwoven here to illustrate similarities and differences in the way Latinos respond and cope with cancer.

As we prepared to write this chapter, we searched the literature, interested to find if the research of others matched our own personal and professional experiences with cancer. However, much of the literature available about caregiving among Latinos describes the experience of those caring for the elderly or for individuals with a mental disorder. Despite a growing trend of multimedia material available that describes how Latinos turn to faith, family, and the power of positive attitude as part of their resources to cope with cancer, for example, *Las Combatientes* [*The Combatants*] (Diaz-Arroyo & Valentin-Lugo, 2004), a movie filmed in Puerto Rico; *Una Etapa Difícil* [*A Difficult Phase*], a book by Mayte Prida (2005); and *Nuestras Historias* [*Our Stories*] (2004), stories of Latina breast cancer survivors; literature about Latino cancer co-survivor experience is scarce.

Research findings suggest, however, the importance of a treatment approach shifting from patient-centered to family-focused (Nijboer, Triemstra, Tempelaar, Sandman, & van den Bos, 1999; Evercare, 2008). The National Alliance for Caregiving (Evercare, 2008) conducted a study that included large representation from areas with the highest concentration of Latino populations in the United States. Findings identified cancer, second to diabetes, among the top health conditions for the need of Latinos to provide informal care at home. Researchers found that most Latino cancer caregivers are young and are mostly women; at least one out of every seven Latino households provides informal caregiving to at least a loved one, and sometimes two. The study also established that Latinos prefer to care for their loved ones at home due to language barriers and distrust of institutions.

A Word or Two about Latinos

Cancer is the second leading cause of death for Latinos (American Cancer Society, 2008). Latinos are also reported to have a lower five-year survival rate from cancer compared to non-Latino whites. Fear and limited access to prevention and early detection services are some of the most significant factors contributing to poor cancer prognosis. In our experience, many— especially younger Latinos—ignore symptoms for a long time, due to fear or lack of health insurance; when they finally find the courage to seek care, it is either too late, or they may require intense or more complex treatment.

There are approximately 400 million Spanish-speaking people around the world. Latinos are the fastest-growing minority group in the United States. By 2050, Latinos are expected to comprise 25% of the U.S. population (U.S. Census Bureau, 2008). The term *Latino* stirs up a significant amount of debate in the United States, beginning almost three decades ago when many were trying to determine the "politically correct" way to address people of Latin descent and most recently due to immigration laws. The debate emerged as the terms *Hispanic vs. Latino* were being explored by the U.S. government as a way to categorize people who spoke Spanish, were born in Latin American countries, or were born in the U.S. to Latin American immigrants. Hispanic was adopted as the official term for census purposes (Shorris, 2001). However, for ease of understanding, this chapter will use the term Latino to refer to individuals from Hispanic or Latino descent.

The Latino ethnic category encompasses people from approximately 26 countries around the world. Latin Americans (people from Central America, South America, and the Spanish-speaking Caribbean) are a product of blended pre-Columbian native Indians, Europeans (Spanish, French, Italian), and Africans brought by settlers to be used as slaves. These rich Latino heritage roots are responsible for marked differences in physical features (e.g., skin color), cultural frames of reference, and linguistic expressions. For example, not all Latinos speak Spanish; some speak French, Portuguese, Creole, or regional dialects.

Diversity among Latinos is demonstrated by differences in educational and socioeconomic backgrounds, diverse views about politics, social status structures, faith, spiritual practices, customs, and beliefs about health and healing. Add to these differences among those who were born and raised in the U.S., and those who moved to the U.S., either at a very young age or later in life—a perspective that considers different levels of acculturation to the U.S. mainstream culture. Such diversity within the "Latino category" poses a great challenge to service providers with limited exposure to or understanding of the Latino mosaic. Many Latinos do not even identify themselves as Latino or Hispanic. Some will argue that they are not Latino but are instead Mexican, Colombian, Spanish, or another specific nationality, and prefer to be addressed as such. Questions about ethnicity or race that appear in questionnaires or medical histories are often confusing to some because in general they do not accurately describe where they are from.

For the most part, while acknowledging differences exist, Latinos are very spiritual and family-oriented; we celebrate life and love to honor our elders, our young, and all in between. We enjoy a passionate discussion about politics, sports, family, or current social affairs, while savoring a good *Café o Te a las 3:00* (coffee or tea at 3:00 P.M.). We often embrace and kiss on the cheek, both when we greet each other and when we say *Nos vemos* or *Hasta Luego* ("so long"). The use of the embrace which can easily be perceived as unprofessional or strange by those who lack understanding of our culture, is a sign of solidarity, compassion, respect, and connection with our own heritage—with what feels closest to home and family.

> *Some of my younger patients greet me and ask for "La Bendición" (a blessing) when they see me. I naturally reply, "Dios me lo bendiga" (God bless you, my child), as I always respond to my children. In conversation with one of my young patients one day, I discovered he perceived me as the closest to his mom for the good care I had provided for him. "She is old and very ill, therefore not able to come to the states to visit me so when I ask for La Bendición, and I receive your blessing, it feels as if it were coming directly from her." (Latina RN)*

Customs such as asking for *La Bendición* from our elders when we greet them or leave their presence, or a kiss on the cheek and the embrace, can be just as therapeutic and healing as the most sophisticated clinical intervention, especially for those with no close relatives in the area—those who are feeling homesick, especially during the initial stages of a cancer diagnosis.

For instance, immigrant Latinos from rural areas (e.g., pueblos or provinces in Mexico) usually live in multigenerational extended family dwellings where they look out for and help each other. They all take part in child care and share a common sense of responsibility for the family well-being. When they move to the United States, they usually reestablish that sense of small town or community by moving to neighborhoods where other relatives or friends from their native areas live.

Who Are the Latino Cancer Co-Survivors?

Many Latinos do not identify with the term co-survivor; we have been socialized to view caregiving as a role expected of us. Many view it as a way to honor our loved ones for all they have done for us. Yet co-survivors are:

* The 67-year-old Puerto Rican main caretaker to her mom with chronic diabetes, who learns as she finishes her breast cancer treatment that her husband of 40 years has lung cancer.
* The 26-year-old sister who just became the main caretaker of older sister diagnosed with endometrial cancer, in addition to becoming the foster mother of her sister's severely developmentally challenged son.
* The 19-year-old who stays at her 21-year-old husband's hospital bedside as they deal with his advanced testicular cancer and provide care for their 6-month-old firstborn.
* The husband who, due to lack of family in the U.S., sends his 34-year-old wife (a stage IV lymphoma patient) and three children back to their native country so the children can adjust to living with the grandmother who will care for them after "Mommy goes to heaven." He remains here to work three jobs so he can support them and afford to call them every day.
* The 23-year-old woman who, in the midst of dealing with her 24-year-old husband's terminal testicular cancer, learns that her mother was diagnosed with breast cancer.
* The young surgeon who copes with her mother's third cancer recurrence, as she establishes her own practice.
* The family that moves to the U.S. seeking the best possible care for their father with advanced prostate cancer.
* Someone's wife, husband, mother, sister . . . someone like you and me.

Contributing factors to Latino co-survivors' stress could be disagreement or discouragement with the treatment choice made by the patient. Caregivers want to be supportive, but sometimes are afraid to voice their opinions, especially if they are young. Their silence is sometimes misinterpreted as lack of interest. Often, the silence could be a sign of lack of understanding, fear, frustration, and powerlessness that can lead to delayed grieving or depression. The high incidence of young adult Latinos diagnosed with cancer has resulted in the phenomenon of teenagers and young adults taking on the caregiving role. An expression commonly heard from young co-survivors:

We accept the role with a positive attitude, others with resignation because that is what is expected of us. Sometimes we have conflicting emotions, because of the Latino value of respect to the family. It is hard to honestly express our opinions. Instead, we do what is expected of us, and sometimes we cannot help it but to be angry and take the anger out on others.

The centrality of family to Latinos places a tremendous amount of pressure on young Latino co-survivors. Family customs hold them accountable for the care of an ill parent or relative, regardless of their own immediate family (e.g., wife, children) and career responsibilities. This unspoken cultural custom is often very difficult for non-Latinos or more acculturated young Latinos to understand—for those who customarily focus first on individual needs and second on the extended family. Co-survivors who belong to blended families may find themselves juggling pressures while trying to be as supportive as possible to their loved one living with cancer. They feel pressured by unrealistic expectations of Latino relatives, coupled with the demands of their non-Latino relatives (e.g., in-laws) who sometimes perceive them as "overinvolved," due to the lack of cultural understanding.

Often, co-survivors get so caught up in their loved one's needs that they do not take the time to care for themselves. Conflicting emotions are not easily verbalized or dealt with due to the Latino value of respect to the family and especially to the elders. Instead, co-survivors do what is expected of them, sometimes becoming isolated, resentful or depressed without access to resources to assist them in processing those feelings. Language barriers make this process even more difficult.

The Initial Diagnosis, Sharing the News, Treatment Decisions

The initial reactions of co-survivors vary based on the stage at which the diagnosis is found: acute, chronic, or advanced (Nijboer et al., 1999; see also chapter 2). Shock, numbness, and fear are the most common reactions to the diagnosis. Subsequently, the patient's loved ones—co-survivors—move into a very active role of taking over new responsibilities such as providing transportation to appointments, figuring out how to access money or some type of insurance to cover the costly cancer treatments, and/or assuming other household responsibilities. When the disease is found at advanced or terminal stage, loved ones usually rally and anchor themselves in either a survivorship or a bereavement mode.

As unbelievable as it may sound, for many Latino cultures—especially those from small towns or provinces with very traditional values—having a disease like cancer is perceived in a fatalistic manner as bad Karma, or as if it is a curse or a punishment from a higher power for something bad they or their ancestors have done. For some indigenous Latin cultures, cancer is perceived as a contagious disease you catch due to "sinful" actions such as living with someone out of wedlock:

> We had to get married through the Church so that she could let go of the idea that her cancer was a punishment from God because we never married after 10 years together. After the wedding her health turned for the worse. She was a candidate for a bone morrow transplant, but her siblings were in Mexico, and we did not have the money to bring them here or to pay for their treatment. Since all of our close family is in Mexico, she went there with our three children. I stayed here to work to support them and send money for her treatments, which are very expensive there. She wanted the children to get used to her mom and sister because they will be in charge of them when she dies.
> (32-year-old husband of Mexican stage IV lymphoma patient)

Many Latino men become very depressed once they learn they have cancer. At times they feel "castrated" by the idea of not being able to provide for their family, or not being able to satisfy their partners sexually:

> My husband clammed up, he was so devastated about not being able to provide for the family, that he did not want to talk about what was happening to him. He did not even want to share it with our closest relatives. I felt I needed to talk about it with others, but respected his position of keeping it to ourselves. I felt we needed to fight this together, but he needed to do it by himself on his own terms. After all, that is what a Latino man does, he takes care of his family. It was really hard to deal with this—we only had each other and our kids, all our family was back in Honduras and we did not want to burden them with our problem. We had been working very hard to send money and help them out.
> (Wife of 39-year-old Honduran, stage III testicular cancer)

Latinos place powerful authority in physicians. Many times people make very important life-altering decisions, such as whether to accept chemotherapy for advanced disease treatment, without a clear understanding of the side effects or the implications these decisions will have in their quality of life. It is important that both survivors and co-survivors learn to use available resources that will help them make informed decisions:

> This illness makes you feel that you lose your roles and self-sufficiency. The doctors, my kids, and my friends made decisions for me. I would have

skipped chemo. I know that if the cancer went to my lungs, there is not much to do. I took the chemo to please my doctor and my family. He [the doctor] is a beautiful person and my family loves me very much. My kids use to tell me you can't give up, Mama . . . you have to keep fighting. In the meantime, my life extinguishes little by little . . . I am too tired to talk or even get up from bed when my grandkids come to visit. I would really enjoy making their favorite dessert. If I didn't have the chemo maybe I could have gone home to my country to visit with relatives that I have not seen in a long time. (67-year-old Peruvian, metastatic lung cancer)

It is important that service providers inform patients about helpful resources, clinical trials, and genetic testing in a linguistically and culturally sensitive way taking into consideration their learning style (e.g., important treatment information is delivered in Spanish by certified translators, not the phone translation lines). Family members, while perhaps available to translate, should not be substitutes for certified translators:

Now that five years have gone by, and my mom is doing well after her breast cancer treatment, I remember that even after all the research I did to get the best possible treatment for her, chills ran down through my spine when I had to translate for the doctors the medical terminology or treatment long term side effects. My mom would say, "Mija, how is that the doctor talked for so long and you translated it just in a few words?" I would explain: it takes longer in English mama. How about the consent forms? I would say to my mom, "Andele firma aqui dice que le va a ir muy bien y que se va a curar" (Sign here; it says you will be fine and it will cure you). I just did not have the heart to tell her all that it said in there. (34-year-old Mexican American co-survivor)

Cancer Is Just Another Thing to Add to the Plate

For some, cancer becomes just another item in their list of life's struggles— one more item among their competing priorities. Many are uninsured or can not afford the deductable or co-payments. Sometimes they are diagnosed with cancer and choose home remedies or faith (they just pray) instead of seeking medical attention—some due to fear of deportation, others due to lack of trust in the medical system based on their or others past negative experiences. Moreover, the current economic recession has left many people without jobs, and a day missed from work equates to a day not paid. Thus some Latinos may feel obligated, despite illness, to work to avoid further economic hardships.

I am still on my chemo. I want to go back to work, but my doctor does not think it is a good idea. Bills are piling up, credit collectors are starting to send nasty letters. We have three children. My wife can only work part-time because we cannot afford child care and most of the time I am too sick to drive myself or the kids. She lost her job because she needed to bring me to my appointments. (34-year-old Peruvian, stage III Hodgkin's lymphoma)

I have to continue working; once my boss finds out I was out because I have testicular cancer and that I am receiving radiation, they will throw me out in a heartbeat. The fact that I am legal does not mean anything to them. Since I work in construction, it becomes a liability for them to have me working 10–12 hours a day under the sun. They are afraid I will get sick and claim workman's compensation, and then it becomes a higher expense for the company. (26-year-old Mexican, stage IV testicular cancer)

Self-reliance and the fear of not wanting to become a burden to others sometimes have a lot to do with how we handle our stress and communicate our needs. Latina women have a tendency to be very stoic and put themselves last when dealing with the physical and emotional side effects of cancer diagnosis and treatments. We know of women who would not attend or who would push back critical follow-up appointments because of family obligations or other priorities. The literature has described this phenomenon as a cultural response to illness. Many times Latinas will neither admit to extreme pain nor ask for assistance, *por no molestar* (so as not to bother):

I am so depressed. I was very active; imagine with five kids ages 6–17. I want to get up and take care of my home and my family but I am so fatigued. The hospital gave me papers to get some help, but I don't really understand what I need to do. My brain is like a fog, and my older kids are so busy going to school, taking care of everything else including the younger ones. I don't want to put another burden on them. I get anxious when friends and family just stop by, as is customary in our counties of origin. I know they have the best intentions, but I feel embarrassed about the conditions of my house. I used to keep my home so nice and clean. Now I do not have the physical strength or "animo" (spirit) to entertain. No, I would never ask for help. It is not in my nature." (41-year-old/ Dominican, stage III Breast Cancer)

Where to Turn: Faith and Family

As Latinos learn about their diagnosis, they usually turn to what they perceive as their immediate sources of support: the strength of faith and family. For most, not different from other ethnic groups, the experience of cancer usually results in a renewed encounter with faith:

When I was diagnosed with my first cancer, it did not affect me as much. I was more focused on the problems I had with my husband. I really did not have too much time to think about my cancer. I used exercise as a way of channeling negative feelings I had about my husband's addiction to drugs. Many thought I was avoiding dealing with my cancer. Little did they know that the stress from the cancer and the treatment were nothing to me compared to the situation at home. Facing cancer a second time was easier, because I have found comfort in my faith and my husband's rehabilitation." (56-year-old Mexican, stage III breast cancer)

The word *family* has a different connotation for Latinos. It means we turn to blood and legal relatives such as husband, wife, sibling, and children. In addition, we turn to *familia postiza* (in-laws and their family). We also turn to the extended family (second, third cousins, people from the neighborhood where we grew up), and we turn to "family by choice." These are individuals with whom by choice we decide to share a significant part of our life's journey; people who by coincidence "moved in and stayed in our hearts," sometimes becoming as close as or even closer than blood relatives—people such as *compadres* (godparents)/close friends, life companions, gay partners, and roommates. Sometimes a coworker or a next-door neighbor becomes the "next of kin" or co-survivor by default because no one else may be available to care for the patient.

However, many experience great despair because they do not want to burden their relatives back home with the "bad news." Many remain silent about their cancer diagnosis and do not share the information until they are done with the treatment or they are close to the end of their lives. Even though family is perceived as a source of support for most, others can perceive family as a source of stress, especially those with strained relationships (Martinez Tyson, 2009). Younger survivors who have been raised in the U.S., and who have established their own independent lives from an early age, have great difficulty adjusting to or depending on relatives for care or emotional or financial support.

Being far away from their family who had remained in their native country is another source of stress. Many feel they have to keep a strong, happy face to avoid burdening or causing worry to their families back home. When the survival rate for their specific type of cancer is low, those with children and no family in the United States worry over what will happen to their children if something happens to them. Others share that while having family come and visit them from their native country is comforting, it is also a source of stress because they feel as if they have to attend to their guests and be a good host, even though they are sick (Martinez Tyson, 2009).

What Works, What Doesn't
Getting used to a new role is a challenge for most people, regardless of their ethnic or cultural background. Becoming "a patient" is very hard, but for some, becoming a caregiver is even harder—we have witnessed survivors trying to be strong and offering support to their co-survivors.

From talking with women over time, we have noticed that when women first learn about their breast cancer diagnosis, there is an increased need for emotional and moral support. Here, a survivor refers to Camp Alegria, a three-day camp found to be effective in educating about cancer and providing emotional support to Latinas (Martinez et al., 2008):

> *When they told me that I had cancer, I felt like dying. I was depressed and didn't want to get out of my house—the hair loss was hard on me. I accepted treatment with resignation, but was sure this cancer would kill me. My family was really busy on their own things; they try to hide their fear by keeping themselves busy. Thanks to Camp Alegria, I met other women that were going through similar situations. Then I joined the LUNA support group. Therefore, my burden was lighter. My support group and the friendships I made at the camp have become part of my family and my desire to keep living.* (71-year-old Puerto Rican, advanced peritoneal stomach cancer)

The need for instrumental support—tangible help—increases as treatment side effects such as limited mobility, nausea, fatigue, aches, and pains arise. However, treatment side effects can last or emerge long after the actual treatment is complete, and thus some women continue to need instrumental support.

Studies report that Latinas are more likely to receive support from other female relatives and *comadres*/close friends (Jones et al., 1999) than from their husbands/partners (Martinez-Schallmoser, Telleen, & MacMullen, 2003). However, while these findings may suggest that women give more support than men, it might be worth considering that husbands and male relatives may be just as supportive, but in modes that are culturally prescribed, such as working to financially support the family and purchasing medications. According to Erwin and colleagues (2005), Latinos have a patriarchal system where sources of power and authority favor the man in male/female relationships and define certain roles and relationships for women. Latino men may be more likely to drive and control access to health care due to their privileged economic status; in addition, Latinas often depend on men financially.

Sometimes relatives move in with the best intentions of providing the most loving care. The task becomes taxing when the patient's or caregiver's idiosyncrasies get in the way and the two cannot reach an agreement (e.g., co-survivor likes to stay busy cleaning and organizing, co-survivor feels the need to control and help). The keys to being an effective co-survivor are flexibility, patience, and recognition of the need for self-care early on. Co-survivors need to allow themselves time to adjust to the new role. Give yourself permission to spend time with other people. Playing it by ear is a good way to go because it also allows the space and the time for your loved one (the patient) to adjust to temporary or permanent loss of his or her roles and independence:

> *I appreciate you bringing me the soup. My son knows that cooking is like a therapy for me, so he touched my heart when he showed up with all the*

ingredients for my favorite soup. I wish I had the energy, but I am not even in the mood to cook. If it wasn't for the soup you brought me, I wouldn't have eaten today. (76-year-old Puerto Rican, third cancer recurrence)

The concept of *presencia* (being present), or having someone in mind, is one of the elements mentioned at support groups as part of healing. *Estar presente* (showing presence) gives Latinos a sense of emotional safety and being able to have *confianza*, or trust in/with someone (Martinez Tyson, 2009). Sharing time and information with others who are going through the same experience is also very effective and helps to keep a positive attitude:

Receiving phone calls, e-mails, text messages, even if brief, were great help. It is hard to call home [Colombia] every day, but just getting an e-mail or a text message saying they are thinking or praying for us was great help. (28-year-old Colombian co-survivor)

Trust and family secrecy issues are some of the factors that interfere the most with Latinos' seeking or accepting counseling as an option. Counseling is also associated with chronic mental illness or an inability to face adversity with *resignación* (resignation), which is what most of us are socialized to do when facing difficult times. Most Latinos, especially those who were raised in more traditional settings, are not open to "counseling." They usually seek assistance with concrete services such as health care coverage, translation of important documents, or some type of help for their loved one. Most do not make appointments and do not like to leave phone messages. This is because some of them come from places where important matters are taken care of in person. For instance, Latinos from the Caribbean call it *las diligencias*—going in person to clarify a billing error or to the bank for transactions.

Latinos may drop by for very concrete issues, but behind those visits there is usually an emotional need they want to address while not in the presence of their loved ones. Sometimes they feel drained by the ongoing demands of the caregiving role, or they are concerned about the patient's lack of progress; their leave from work is about to end and their family member still requires round-the-clock attention. In order to engage in counseling, they need to perceive the counselor as part of their inner circle or their extended family. One solution is to allow for *familismo* (sense of family) to take place.

This can be frustrating if working in a fast-paced cancer center, but we have learned to schedule appointments far apart and to allow some flexibility for those interruptions. Latino patients usually do not want to sit in the office for a "counseling session," but they welcome a short *platica or conversación* (brief conversation) while sipping a cup of coffee or tea. In our center, Latinos are more comfortable sitting in the library or the break room—both have round tables that resemble a home kitchen table. The kitchen or dining area is where the heart of many Latino families resides— it is, for most, where important conversations or decisions take place. For our support group meetings, we arrange several small conference room tables to simulate a large dining room table. We sit around the table—there is always some food to share, and it feels like a large family *convive* (a word used by Mexicans to describe a family gathering to share a special time).

Many times caregivers or family members ask, "How are you doing or feeling?" and do not get a true answer; if they do, it is not an elaborate one. This is problematic, as communication is a two-way street. For example, a cancer survivor can say "just fine" or "so-so," and the caregiver can say "okay" and move on with his or her day. Caregivers can probe further to determine how they can help the cancer survivor feel better, or what can be done around the house to lessen the cancer survivor's daily burden. Cancer survivors can help caregivers by verbalizing their needs.

What else works? Listening to music, watching a *telenovela* (soap opera), reminiscing about good memories, and simply finding humor in the most ordinary moments. Building memories that will transcend time and space—reminders of the special time you and your loved one spent together working toward a common goal: your loved one's comfort and your peace of mind.

About Closing Chapters and New Beginnings

For most Latinos, cancer provides an opportunity to continue working on the resiliency they have developed through dealing with prior adversities and traumas. For the most part, Latinos view their cancer experience as a positive life-altering experience when they take the opportunity to integrate healthy changes into their lifestyles. Life and living take on a totally different meaning.

After an intense time at your loved one's side, there will be a period of transition during which you and your loved one will adjust to life after cancer treatment. As with many other changes in life, this will also bring some anxieties and uncertainties—new lessons to learn. Patience and being gentle on yourself will be key. At the initial signs of your loved one's progress with treatment, it is okay for you to transition back into your daily life routine as it was before cancer moved in. This will allow your loved one, the survivor, to also begin finding his or her "new self after cancer."

Recommendations for Co-Survivors

1. Actively listen with your heart to the unspoken needs of your loved one, and clearly communicate your needs.
2. You probably will not get a true response if you ask, "How are you today?" Instead, ask, "What were the highlights of your day today?"
3. Ask for help or accept assistance from family and friends early on. Not addressing your needs may lead to burnout and resentment. It is okay to say no, or to buy yourself some time, by saying "Let me think about it and I'll get back to you" when dealing with others' expectations of your time and attention. Co-survivors need to keep their feelings in check. Communicate your needs openly and with

respect. Be flexible. Your loved one may have a different perspective, or may just like to do things in a different way.

4. If you see your loved one is not getting the care he or she deserves, address it with the hospital management.

5. When possible, find a doctor or facility that can best address the needs of both you and your loved one; it is your right.

6. Consider that others may feel just as powerless as you do and want so much to help out, but do not know how. Make a list of future engagements or holidays when you need help. For example, if you are usually the cook or host, it is okay to have someone else coordinate and host the next family gathering.

7. Make a list, with the survivor's input, of things that need to be done or are coming up, and keep it handy for when someone asks, "What can I do to help?"

8. It is okay to take a break from the front line to recharge your energy. It is okay to exercise, clean, listen to music, grieve, or simply do nothing at all.

9. Take time to laugh and build memorable moments. Take pictures of special moments and happy occasions. Laughing is good therapy for you and for your loved one.

10. Take on a new hobby or practice, such as meditation, yoga, or guided imagery.

Recommendations for Health Care Providers

1. Probe patients and their families understanding of diagnostic information and treatment choices they are making. Start by trying to establish good rapport. Try to greet Latino patients in Spanish. (A physician saying *"Hola"* (Hi) and genuinely smiling, showing concern to a Latino patient, turns a communication challenge into a much more manageable encounter.) In general, Latinos are very warmhearted people and truly appreciate it when others reach out to them.

2. Respect cultural norms and beliefs regarding a Latina patient's choice to disclose, or not, her cancer diagnosis, personal worries, and concerns to her family.

3. Understand the added burden and stress cancer may cause *immigrant* Latina cancer patients and the availability of their social support.

4. Do a brief cultural assessment to determine level of acculturation by asking "What is your country of origin?" or "How long have you been in the U.S.?" (Do not assume that every Latino is Puerto Rican or Mexican.)

5. When possible, allow people the time and space to express their feelings and carry out their religious rituals.

6. Do not assume Latinos are noncompliant. Many other family and life issues may have high priority in their lives and affect their ability to follow through with treatment.

7. Educate family and caregivers about the short- and long-term physical and psychosocial effects of cancer and its treatment. Teach them about cancer patients' needs so they may better understand what their loved ones are experiencing. Family members may learn what they can do to be supportive without patients feeling as though they are burdening their families or putting their own needs before their families' needs.

8. Reach out to give special attention to Latino cancer patients who have immigrated to the U.S. alone. These patients usually have the least support and are often most vulnerable to stressors. Recognize that regardless of time in the U.S., Latino immigrants maintain close ties and frequently communicate with family and friends in their native countries. Enabling Latino immigrants (e.g., providing calling cards) to communicate with family and friends during cancer treatment(s) might prove a way of providing support.

9. Be aware of the importance of establishing relationships and building rapport when working with vulnerable or underserved populations. This may involve a lot of personal time and outreach.

10. Consider verbal and nonverbal forms of communication when developing support programs for Latinos.

11. Do not make assumptions of language proficiency or education level just because of a Spanish surname. Provide patient education and information in the patient's language. This may entail having translators for patients who speak little English, especially in an oncology setting, where medical jargon and complex terms are often used to explain and describe treatment plans. Spanish-speaking patients should be offered an interpreter, even if they speak a little English and feel they can get by with their level of proficiency. Providers are one of the main sources of informational support for cancer patients, and thus it is crucial that patients and co-survivors are able to understand and communicate effectively with their doctors.

12. Use bilingual and bicultural translation service providers when possible; a translation line is to be used for short conversations. It should not be used to share diagnostic or prognosis information.

Personal Reflections from the Authors

Mother's Day, 2009. I pick up the phone and listen to a message from a woman who did not bear any children, but who has been like a mother to many, especially to me. She said her customary greetings and then paused. "I have sort of bad news . . . pancreatic cancer, very aggressive. I have decided not to do anything and enjoy the days I have left with the best possible quality of life. I needed to be the one to let you know." She is one of my mentors and one of the most influential people in my life; the person who opened the doors for me to enter graduate school 25 years ago and to whom I owe much of the person and the professional I am today.

I spent the rest of the morning in shock: speechless, numb, in disbelief. Sadness settled in . . . despair . . . kind of a twilight zone that sucks you in, leaving you with no sense of direction and feeling very isolated, even in a room full of people. I called other loved ones, hoping they could wake me up from the bad dream. They reacted the same way I did and understood exactly how I felt. Personally and professionally I have faced many losses in the past, and the initial reaction always seems to be the same. I imagine you have felt the same way at some point in your life. A good starting point for co-survivors is to seek comfort in sharing with people who are part of our inner circle.

* * *

I have faced several challenges during the course of my research and work with Latina cancer survivors. After hearing their personal struggles, I felt it was my duty to advocate for them and make an extra effort to connect them to local resources and find information for them. I heard the fear and desperation in their voices. I could not begin to imagine how it feels to know you have cancer and to have to wait weeks to find a doctor or facility to receive treatment. The fact that I was working at a well-known cancer institute made it even more frustrating to me. Through my volunteer work as LUNA support group facilitator, I developed personal relationships with some of the survivors and their families, which have enriched my life. Now, my new position as a researcher at a cancer research center and my years of participation in the cancer biomedical multidisciplinary community network have equipped me to advocate for Latinas. I use my position as a vehicle to open doors and be part of organizational changes that allow Latinos access to care, genetic research, and clinical trials. This is my way of co-surviving and showing *presencia*—being present.

* * *

Cancer is a personal battle, and we as co-survivors need to understand that it is not a battle that we can fight on our own—we can help by providing love, a listening heart, and the tools that our loved ones or patients need to continue their journey. Working in cancer as a health care executive has been a very rewarding, but challenging, experience for me. I am challenged with many difficult cases of uninsured patients that want a different course of treatment, that are depressed, that have unresolved issues with their relatives, and come to us for advice or interventions. . . . The words faith and hope are really important; because of my faith, I look at life, illnesses, and death in a different way. I am driven to implement processes and programs to specifically address the needs of the underserved and for those with the least resources. I have made my line of work an instrument of peace and a way of opening new opportunities to lessen the stress for all patients with whom I come into contact on a daily basis.

* * *

I was 18 years old and just started my first year of college when I learned my grandmother was diagnosed with cancer. This news was shocking, but I did not get sad or cry. I assumed she would get the appropriate care she needed and that in a few weeks she would be okay. I buried myself in my studies and joined several school extracurricular activities for distraction. It was my way of coping. My caretaking role was, for the most part, from a distance. I would help translate often complex and critical medical documents, for many of which I guessed the intended meaning. The times I accompanied her to doctor and hospital visits, clinical staff would put me in the difficult role of the medical interpreter. I struggled to find the right words to express what my grandmother was feeling or what the doctor was telling me without losing the appropriate meaning. As the only person from the family who was attending "college," I was also looked upon to make difficult decisions such as hospice care and funeral arrangements, which I was not emotionally ready to face.

After my grandmother's passing, I regretted my avoidant behavior and missed the moments I should have spent with her. Now that years have passed and I have more experience with cancer from my various community involvements, academic activities, and life experience, I learned that my coping mechanism was not healthy for me and my family. I should have asked for help and sought comfort from other young co-survivors. I should also have told the clinical staff that I needed help with translation and required a medical translator. These actions would have better prepared me to deal with my grandmother's illness and cope with the side effects she had; I wish I would have been more informed. The wisdom I gained from my young adulthood experience with cancer helped with my husband's recent cancer diagnosis. The love and support I received from my fellow peers and others going through similar experiences allowed me to co-survive more effectively and provide better care to my husband.

Alma, Dina, Gloria, and Claudia

References

American Cancer Society. (2008). *Cancer facts & figures for Hispanics/Latinos 2006–2008*.

Erwin, D. O., Johnson, V. A., Feliciano-Libid, L., Zamora, D., & Jandorf, L. (2005). Incorporating cultural constructs and demographic diversity in the research and development of a Latina breast and cervical cancer education program. *Journal of Cancer Education, 20*(1), 39–44.

Díaz-Arroyo, A. & Valentín-Lugo, S. (Producers), & Valentín-Lugo, S. (Director). (2004). Las Combatientes [The Combatants] [Motion picture]. Puerto Rico: Producciones Copelar.

Evercare® study of Hispanic family caregiving in the U.S.: Findings from a national study. (2008). Minnetonka, MN: Evercare and Bethesda, MD: National Alliance for Caregiving.

Jones, L. A., Hajek, R., Chilton, J. A., Esparza, A., Garza, S. A. G., & Gonzalez, R., et al. (1999). Implementing effective recruitment strategies for a cancer-prevention trial in older Hispanic women: A clinical trial model. In D. Weiner (Ed.), *Preventing and controlling cancer in North America: A cross-cultural perspective*. Westport, CT: Praeger.

Martinez, D., Aguado Loi, C. X., Martinez, M. M., Flores, A. E., & Meade, C. D. (2008). Development of a cancer camp for adult Spanish-speaking survivors: Lessons learned from Camp Alegria. *Journal of Cancer Education, 23*(1), 4–9.

Martinez-Schallmoser, L., Telleen, S., & MacMullen, N. J. (2003). The effect of social support and acculturation on postpartum depression in Mexican American women. *Journal of Transcultural Nursing, 14*(4), 329–338.

Martinez Tyson, D. (2009). *The social context of stress and social support among immigrant Latinas diagnosed with breast cancer*. Unpublished doctoral dissertation, University of South Florida, Tampa.

Nijboer, C., Triemstra, M., Tempelaar, R., Sandman, R., & van den Bos, G. A. M. (1999). Determinants of caregiving experiences and mental health of partners of cancer patients. *Cancer, 86*, 577–588.

Nuestras historias: Mujeres Hispanas sobreviendo el cancer del seno/Our stories: Hispanic women surviving breast cancer. A publication of *Redes En Acción*: The National Hispanic/Latino Cancer Network; National Cancer Institute Grant No. U0 1 CA 86117-01 (D. Presswood, ed.). San Antonio: Quadrangle Press, Inc. Available online at http://www.redesenaccion.org/historias_bk.html.

Prida, M. (2005). *Una etapa difícil: Mi lucha contra el cancer* [A difficult phase: My battle against cancer]. Miami, FL: Planeta. (First published in 2002 by Terra Entertainment, Los Angeles.)

Shorris, E. (2001). *Latinos: A biography of the people*. New York: W. W. Norton

U.S. Census Bureau (2008). Hispanic population of the United States. Date retrieved: June 01, 2009. Retrieved from http://www.census.gov/population/www/socdemo/hispanic/hispanic.html.

Coping in a Gay, Lesbian, Bisexual, and Transgendered Family

We Are Family: Coping with Cancer in the Gay, Lesbian, Bisexual, Transgendered Community

Sarah Sample

NURSE: "Is your family coming to visit?"

FEMALE PATIENT: "My family is here! She's been here every day since I was admitted. Judy is sitting by the window—she is my life partner."

Later, in conversation with social worker:

FEMALE PATIENT: "I remember filling out the forms for admission and arguing with a clerk that I am closer to my partner than I am to my mother—that Judy is my next of kin, and who I trust to make decisions for me if I can't. In the end, I was too overwhelmed by my fears of the surgery and of having cancer to press the point. Later, during recovery in the hospital, I kept being asked by nurses and aides if Judy was my sister, or my daughter."

The above scenario is not unusual for Lesbian/Gay/Bisexual/Transgendered (LGBT) families. As in heterosexual families, stresses and uncertainties throughout the cancer journey can impact in many ways, depending on family stories, socioeconomic status, culture, ethnicity, and gender differences.

LGBT families are as diverse as heterosexual families. In its broadest sense, family is composed of people who have a shared history and a shared future. LGBT families may comprise a single parent, blended families, multiple generations, a couple with or without children, and many other variations. Just like heterosexual families, we are family.

However, many issues specific to LGBT families are not addressed in mainstream health care systems. The assumption of heterosexuality, and the negative repercussions following disclosure of one's sexual orientation, are challenges to the LGBT population. The ability to cope with stressors associated with a cancer diagnosis is compounded by the homophobia of others and their assumption of heterosexuality. Homophobia is usually defined as the irrational fear of, aversion to, or discrimination against the LGBT population. Internalized homophobia is when an LGBT person accepts society's stereotypes and negative labels, and then applies them to her- or himself.

Dr. Kate O'Hanlan, a gynecologic surgical oncologist, past president of the American Gay and Lesbian Medical Association, and co-author of a medical report called "Homophobia as a Health Hazard," educates the medical community and the general public on LGBT health issues. Dr. O'Hanlan states that being gay or lesbian is not inherently hazardous, but some risk factors are conferred through "homophobic fallout" (O'Hanlan, 2001). Homophobia fallout increases health risks and barriers to care because the LGBT community is either hesitant or reluctant to approach health systems.

The health risks and barriers to care that increase cancer risks in the LGBT population include less childbearing or late-in-life childbirth, high body mass index (BMI), smoking, alcohol abuse, and medical care avoidance (O'Hanlan, 2001). Again, many in the LGBT population are afraid to "come out" to their health care providers because of either perceived or direct experience of homophobic attitudes (Fobair et al., 2001). Members of the LGBT population are more reluctant to seek health care due to fears of how they will be treated. The implications of avoiding the health care system can be serious.

By avoiding routine doctor visits, one is less likely to undergo screening tests for cancers, such as mammograms, pap tests, and PSA levels. Lower screening rates compared to the general population can result in a later diagnosis or a diagnosis of advanced cancer, leading to increased mortality rates. Although times have changed somewhat in medical settings, the LGBT population can still be rendered invisible by assumptions based on perceptions of sexual orientation and gender. One woman reported having to tell the nurse at her oncologist's office multiple times that *her partner* was there with her, not her friend. Often, LGBT patients are asked when they last had intercourse. Some lesbians have never had intercourse. If LGBT people do come out, it may be assumed that they don't have family and that they lead unhealthy lifestyles.

Coping with legal issues surrounding cancer is still a challenge for the LGBT population. Non-recognition of LGBT relationships and family can create obstacles—particularly surrounding end-of-life concerns. It is important for the family to have legal documents such as wills, power of attorney, advance care plans, and cohabitation agreements, and for these documents to be explicit. Fortunately, many insurance companies and employers are recognizing LGBT couples and families. In Canada, for instance, marriage is legal. Health care benefits for same sex couples are available in most provinces and territories in Canada.

In this chapter, I primarily address lesbian and bisexual female families coping with cancer, as I have had less direct experience in my clinical oncology work with gay/bisexual men and transgendered people. Little research has been published on the experience of individuals living with cancer in the LGBT community, and even less addressing LGBT families. Anecdotally, we know LGBT families cope like any other families, but homophobia can compound problems and complicate the cancer experience. Lesbians and gay men approach the world differently as an invisible minority.

On Coming Out—How Did I Get Here?

In my practice at the cancer clinic, I have met numerous lesbians and gay people and their partners living with cancer. Many women have told me that they specifically seek me out as a lesbian social worker because it is safe for them. Some say they are managing on their own, but are relieved to know that I am there if they do need support in the future. A young gay man expressed his relief when he became aware that I am a lesbian and began to open up and express his deepest fears. Some want information about practical and financial concerns. Others are looking for support surrounding fears and worries about cancer spreading, fear of dying, and relationship concerns—the same concerns that bring all other people to seek support and counseling to cope with cancer.

I stood in front of a women's breast cancer support group in an affluent neighborhood in the city where I work to give a talk about lesbians living with cancer. I was nervous, but not because I was giving a public talk. Normally, I am comfortable in front of an audience if I know my topic, but the subject I was about to discuss involved my being public about my sexual orientation. The majority of women in this group were white, heterosexual, and middle class; I was afraid I would not be accepted. I felt this was in part due to my internalized homophobia. I asked myself, "How did I get here?"

Well, I happened to be on a planning committee for a conference on breast cancer. When we were asked for ideas for breakout sessions, I suggested a panel on lesbians and breast cancer. This suggestion came from my experience the previous year facilitating the Lesbian/Bisexual/Transgendered (LBT) women's group at the Cancer Centre. There was a moment of silence at the planning meeting. Then one of the physicians asked why a panel would be necessary because she didn't see any difference between a heterosexual and a homosexual breast. I replied that the very reason there needed to be a panel about lesbians and breast cancer was because that question was asked. To the physician's credit, she thought about what I said and called me the next day to ask me to give a talk to her local breast cancer support group.

The night of the presentation, I began my talk with a few questions. Do you remember when you were first diagnosed? Do you recall deciding whom you were going to tell and when and how you were going to tell them? Do you remember how you felt? Were you anxious about how your family and friends would respond to your diagnosis? Did you wonder about what the consequences of telling them might be? All the women in that room were nodding back at me. Yes, they did remember the awkwardness, the anxiety and fears about whom and when to tell, and if that would impact their relationships with friends and family. And then I asked them to imagine having to do that your whole life on a regular basis. Responses were overwhelming. They got it. They began to understand the fears and anxiety surrounding "coming out" about sexual orientation.

Coming out is about acknowledging same sex preference to yourself and to others. It is a lifelong process. You continually assess whom to come out to, when to come out to someone, and how to do it. The process of coming out is impacted by social norms and assumptions, many of which are heterosexist and homophobic. This is compounded by an internalized homophobia developed by the experience of living in a perceived homophobic society. Coming out is a deeply personal and emotional activity and can be a profoundly life-altering act. Some may never come out—living in a state suspended between the homosexual world and the heterosexual world.

An Example LBT Cancer Support Program

In a Canadian study (Katz, 2009), lesbian and gay participants identified as a concern the lack of cancer support groups in their community. As one example of what is possible at the British Columbia Cancer Centre, the LBT cancer support program began as a pilot project in 1998 in response to requests by a number of lesbian patients. The women expressed the need for emotional support in coping with cancer and responding to homophobic attitudes.

I hesitated in starting the group at the cancer clinic because of my own fears of coming out in a medical setting. I was afraid of what the consequences of coming out would be for my career and my work relationships. However, I was convinced to do so when one lesbian said, "It is hard enough to face cancer without simultaneously worrying about coming out to my health care provider and how that might affect the care that I receive." In a safe, accepting, and supportive group environment, the women have been able to talk openly about their lives and how cancer affects their families. Their comments include:

> *I have not experienced overt discrimination, but I have certainly felt my sexual preference to be invisible, although I have always been very open about it. Too often my partner was referred to as my sister or friend. I feel*

strongly that the work of making resources available to lesbians should not be left up to one or two staff members who may be lesbians. I see this as an example of institutionalized homophobia.

The support group is a place to touch feelings not otherwise explored. It's a safe place to discuss common concerns about cancer without having to explain or worry about homophobia from other group members, or facilitators. In other support groups, I did not feel comfortable raising so-called "lesbian issues."

Sometimes, the number of group attendees is large enough to split the group in two—one group for patients and one for partners/support people. This gives each group an opportunity to express their fears and concerns. Like heterosexual couples, the women couples wanted to protect each other from sad feelings, fear, or anger. The women in the LBT group were explicit about the difference in this group apart from other cancer support groups. They felt safer talking about their range of issues with other lesbians, knowing they would not be subjected to any homophobic responses.

The lack of emotional safety lesbians felt within the larger institution underlies the importance of having their own support group. Safety is one of the essential ingredients of any support group—to be able to express oneself without fearing consequences. A woman in the support group relates:

There are concerns that are specific to lesbians that I only feel comfortable to discuss with other lesbians—for example, impact on relationships, roles, financial concerns, family conflict, and having one's partner acknowledged as next of kin.

Another woman states:

I attended an earlier support group for support people whose family and/ or friends had cancer, and had to go through the stressful process of coming out in order to be able to talk about supporting my same sex partner who has breast cancer. A lot of my energy in the group was involved with fears around homophobia, even though the facilitators were excellent and accepting, as was most of the group.

From my experience in the lesbian/bisexual support group, the lesbian partners of women with cancer often have more difficulty coping and have fewer support programs available to them than do heterosexual partners. For instance, one of the women in the LBT group, a breast cancer patient, joined a dragon boat team. Her partner supported her by attending races and social functions along with other spouses. All of the other partners were men, and she didn't feel comfortable being part of this men's "group." While there is some recognition in the cancer community that male partners of women living with cancer need support, there is really very little acknowledgment that the lesbian has a partner, let alone that she also needs support.

Some LGBT couples have little or no family support from their family of origin or extended family. One woman stated, "Sometimes you come out and your family disowns you. And if you get cancer, it's not like you have your mother and your sister and your family around to support you, so you really need to find a community of friends." However, a cancer diagnosis can lead to a reevaluation of the family of origin relationships and sometimes force discussion with family of origin about sexual orientation. This may lead to resolution of old conflicts.

Creating a "Family of Choice"

The lack of support for LGBT people with cancer who are geographically isolated is also of concern (Sinding, Grassau, & Barnoff, 2006). Through the Wellness Community, online support groups are now offered for patients, family, and caregivers throughout North America. The real-time weekly groups are facilitated by specifically trained professionals. Online support is especially advantageous for people who are isolated. They may live in rural areas or be unable to attend a support group because of taking care of loved ones. Online support specifically for the LGBT community could be particularly helpful for isolated LGBT people who are unlikely to be able to pull together a support group in their small town or are reluctant to "come out."

There can be benefits to being part of the LGBT community. Many lesbians living with cancer view their friends, the lesbian community, and sometimes ex-partners as family—creating a "family of choice." By calling on family of choice, communities of support can be quickly formed: rides to medical appointments are arranged, meals are organized, and child care is offered. These support networks are generally reliable and very effective. Research shows that lesbians are more likely than heterosexual women to report receiving support from their friends. A study by Fobair et al. (2001) found that lesbians with cancer experienced more help with practical tasks from their partners and felt more listened to, cared for, and loved than heterosexual women.

Dyson (2004) explored the experiences of five lesbians diagnosed with cancer, looking at how their individual support network, or community of predominantly lesbians, came together to provide emotional and practical support following a cancer diagnosis. Although trauma is considered to have negative consequences, Dyson argued that facing adverse situations can also lead to psychological growth, and found that the mobilization of the women's community became a factor in posttraumatic growth. That is, the support of community served as a catalyst for individual growth for the participants—including a strengthening of relationships, new appreciation of life, and new potential for themselves. Felicia's story shows how community came together to provide support and how she has grown from her experience.

Case Example: Felicia's Story. Felicia is a 51-year-old lesbian living with recurrent and metastatic cancer of the appendix. She was diagnosed when she was 39. As Felicia's family of origin did not live nearby, her lesbian and gay friends came to her aid. At one point when she was in the hospital and it seemed that she was nearing the end of her life, her community organized meetings to

* assist in discharge planning
* set up an online calendar schedule for spending time with Felicia
* assist with injections
* bring in meals
* take her to medical appointments.

Felicia's community, or "family of choice," made sure that she was seldom alone after she voiced fears and concerns about being alone. Fortunately, Felicia's health has improved since that time and she continues to live her life as fully as possible while still undergoing chemotherapy when necessary. She has made incredible progress through individual and group counseling and now says she wants to have fun—she lives as if there is no tomorrow! Felicia is confident that if she is sick again, her community will be there, and she knows that she will be cared for.

At the cancer clinic in British Columbia where I founded the LBT support group, gay men and transgendered men and women have inquired about a support group for themselves. Unfortunately, I have to tell them that at this point there isn't one, and I am not aware of any in the community. I feel particularly sad about a gay male couple who lived in the suburbs and had little support. They had no biological family and few friends. Because they lived outside the urban area, they were not connected with the gay community. The only emotional and practical support they received was from a heterosexual couple that lived nearby. A couple of transgendered women (transitioned male to female) inquired about attending the LBT support group. One of them came once and didn't return. The other decided that it wouldn't be helpful, as she thought she would be more comfortable in a group of transgendered women. Isolation is a significant experience with gay men and transgendered individuals, but can be addressed as seen in Kevin and Arnold's story.

Case Example: Kevin and Arnold's Story. Kevin is young, a 21-year-old man from Brazil who has lived with his common-law partner, Arnold, for almost two years. He was in the process of immigrating and continuing school when he was diagnosed with osteosarcoma of the left pelvis. Kevin was admitted to the cancer hospital on an urgent basis. Arnold knew that he would have to present himself as Kevin's husband in order to stay with him in the hospital, and advocate for Kevin throughout the cancer journey—the consequences of *not* coming out to the medical professionals outweighed his fears of coming out.

Before the cancer diagnosis, both men were only out to their mothers. For instance, at work, the only person Arnold had told was his boss. After Kevin's diagnosis, it was a gradual and thoughtful process, for Arnold especially, to come out to the rest of his family and friends. Although he was fearful of coming out, Arnold expressed relief when no one turned away from him and Kevin. Medical professionals and friends have been supportive and nonjudgmental of their relationship.

Kevin's mother traveled from Brazil and moved in with the couple. Kevin explained that his mother would not likely have come if his partner had been female—his mother would have assumed that he was being taken care of. Kevin's mother now sees that her son is loved and cared for by Arnold. Both feel supported by their mothers and a few close friends.

During Kevin's treatment, one thing that angered Arnold was that they were *not* told that chemotherapy could cause infertility. The couple had planned to have children and would have liked to have been asked if they wished to be directed to a sperm clinic. They wondered if the doctors did not ask them about family plans because the couple is gay.

Kevin and Arnold recently attended a young adult cancer retreat. Kevin expressed relief that he had the opportunity to talk about the isolation he felt by being gay in a heterosexual world. Both men expressed how they felt loved and accepted by the young adult cancer group where they found connection and felt less isolated. The connection with other young adults has given them strength, hope, and courage to cope with a future of uncertainty. Kevin and Arnold discovered that receiving support from those who accept them for who they are was most important and that it did not necessarily have to come from the gay and lesbian community.

Although society, especially in urban centers, is generally more accepting of LGBT individuals, homophobia and discrimination still prevail in health care settings. Many LGBT people are still afraid to come out to their healthcare providers. We experience higher levels of stress, reduced social support from family of origin, and a strained relationship with the health care system (Fobair et al., 2001).

At a recent Lesbian Cancer Forum in Vancouver, British Columbia, a 52-year-old woman, recently diagnosed with breast cancer, told a keynote speaker—her own oncologist—that she previously had been afraid to come out to her. She had been reluctant to come out to her oncologist out of apprehension and fear of any consequences to her treatment and care. Despite the oncologist's having never given this woman any indication that she would receive adverse care because of her sexual orientation, the woman was still afraid to be honest about her supports, life, and community. In order to best support any patient and their loved ones, mindfulness of negative and positive repercussions of how they live their life is essential.

LGBT families cope with a cancer diagnosis like most families. However, interrelated issues involving the assumption of heterosexuality, negative impact of self-disclosure, and internalized homophobia compound the experience of living with a life-threatening illness such as cancer. Cultural stigma and barriers to care may increase physical, mental, and emotional risk to health in LGBT families. Although such realities within the LGBT community can lend themselves to greater burdens and challenges during a time of life that is already wrought with stress, such marginalization for many has also provided fertile ground for a strong community to take root.

References

Dyson, T. (2004). *Lesbians with cancer: Community and posttraumatic growth.* Unpublished master's thesis, University of British Columbia, Vancouver, British Columbia, Canada.

Fobair, P., O'Hanlan, K., Koopman, C., Classen, C., Dimiceli, S., Drooker, N., et al. (2001). Comparison of lesbian and heterosexual women's response to newly diagnosed breast cancer. *Psycho-Oncology, 10*(1), 40–51.

Katz, A. (2009). Gay and lesbian patients with cancer. *Oncology Nursing Forum, 36*(2), 203–207.

O'Hanlan, K. A. (2001). Homophobia as a health hazard: Report of the gay and lesbian medical association. Retrieved September 1, 2009, from http://ohanlan.com/phobiahzd.htm

Sinding C., Grassau, P., & Barnoff, L. (2006). Community support, community values: The experiences of lesbians diagnosed with cancer. *Women & Health, 44*(2), 59–79.

PART 2

FURTHER SUPPORT AND OPTIONS

CHAPTER 11

Finding Support through Use of the Internet

Ilkka Saarnio, with Lorraine Johnston

I f you have cancer, you need people around you. The Internet can help you. I am a 64-year-old retired engineer living in Tampere, Finland. Tampere is on the latitude of Anchorage; as there, the winters in Tampere are usually cold but bearable, and the summers mild and sunny (that is, if global warming doesn't ruin the whole system). I was diagnosed with a non-Hodgkin's lymphoma (NHL) in February 1995. I was in shock, which I imagine is the first reaction of everyone in a similar situation. Doubtfulness prevailed. I had good friends around me, but they didn't know how to behave or what to say. So they did not do or say much—you find that in Finland. The doctor said that my type of NHL was one that, as yet, no one had been cured of entirely.

When I could breathe, I tried to find information. In 1995, the Internet was still young, but somehow I found a link to the HEM-ONC listserv. HEM-ONC was, and still is, "an unmoderated discussion list for patients, family, friends, researchers, and physicians, to discuss clinical and non-clinical issues and advances pertaining to Leukemia, Lymphoma and Multiple Myeloma. It includes patient experiences, psychosocial issues, new research, clinical trials, and discussions of current treatment practices and alternatives. The principal focus is expected to be information and reassurance for patients and loved ones" (http://acor.org/leukemia/cll/hemonc.html).

On HEM-ONC, you registered, introduced yourself, and started to "talk." In my experience, there were people who remained in the background, just following the discussion. The discussion was lively. But when you came out with your story, there were always responses: advice or information from a doctor or someone with knowledge or experience; a comforting word; or an expression of empathy or interest.

Over time, you came to know the people on the listserv. You experienced their ups and downs, lived through the stem cell transplantation process of the young daughter in a family, and finally participated in their joy when the donor met the family. You followed the medical studies of a young man and saw how he got wiser and finally graduated as a doctor with a special interest in cancer. You joined in the congratulations.

In my experience, the doctors involved with the Internet site seemed to be dedicated to serving the listserv members. They answered all our questions in an understandable way. There were people who knew everything about hematological cancers, and if they didn't know the answers, they found out. Two of these special—and central—persons were GrannyBarb (http://cll.acor.org/GrannyBarb.htm) and Lorraine, both prepared to help anyone. When I posted my story on the site, I was fortunate to be adopted by GrannyBarb and Lorraine—both living in the United States while I lived in Finland. GrannyBarb was a leukemia survivor and the list manager, Lorraine the wife of a Hodgkin's survivor. A friendship developed among us, and we began to e-mail each other outside the listserv. This kind of friendship was new to me. I learned a lot about their families. I could "speak" to them about my daily life and happenings and all the troubles and feelings created by the cancer and the chemotherapy. There was no feeling of overloading them.

I was careful in talking with people close to me at home, thinking that I had to spare them from excessive worry. Quite simply, GrannyBarb and Lorraine were a lifeline, and they kept me alive. I could openly tell them the good and bad feelings; they responded with empathy, understanding, and support. My NHL was treated for two years. During that time, our messages changed from outpourings of sadness, worry, and problems to updates about my life and health in general. GrannyBarb and Lorraine had a delicious sense of humor, and their messages enlightened my day.

As an engineer, my work was in assistive technology for the elderly and for people with disabilities. I used to travel to the United States annually to attend conferences of the Rehabilitation Engineering and Assistive Technology Society of North America (RESNA). I spoke with GrannyBarb a few times on the phone during my visits. Worrying news came in 2003 about the return of her leukemia. GrannyBarb passed away in June 2003, leaving behind sorrow but also gratitude for what she had done by helping others.

When you lose a friend, you need an opportunity to say good-bye. That feeling—a need to say good-bye—remained with me. GrannyBarb had lived in St. Louis, Missouri. The RESNA Conference in Washington, DC, in 2008 would take me closer to St. Louis than I had ever been before. Using the Internet, Lorraine helped me to find the cemetery in St. Louis where GrannyBarb was buried.

I reserved six days after the conference to drive a rental car to St. Louis and back. I had the address of the cemetery and printouts of Google maps for navigation. St. Louis was farther away from Washington than I anticipated, but I did find the cemetery. A very kind cemetery director told me that GrannyBarb had been cremated. He guided me to her niche in the mausoleum—a beautiful place where I sat down at peace. I said good-bye to GrannyBarb and told her of my gratitude for her friendship. The farewell was a calming experience for me.

Driving to St. Louis and back showed me a good slice of America. There was time to listen to the radio, learn about politics, and understand the differences between ash and maple as materials for baseball bats. I learned that American motels are exactly as seen in the movies. I enjoyed that trip.

In December 2004, I was diagnosed with prostate cancer. It was advanced, so no radical treatment was suggested. Instead, I started hormone therapy. I tried to learn as much information as possible from the Internet, but this time, instead of looking for a discussion group, I went to the local cancer association in Tampere in search of a peer support group. I found that what happens is the same as on the Internet: discussions, sharing experiences, having the opportunity to talk about one's own feelings, and support from the experts. The only difference was face-to-face discussions.

If I hadn't found this group, I would certainly have looked for an Internet group. On the Internet, you can find every possible type of information you need. Doctors don't seem to be angry if you refer during your visit to something you saw on the Web. There are now hundreds of cancer fora on the Internet. Some threads are quite short—for instance, fewer than 10 responses—but there are sometimes threads that last several months. Discussions are mostly about peer support, experiences, stories, and encouragement. Thanks to the Internet, the possibility of finding a support group has increased tenfold.

CHAPTER 12

Finding Funds to Help with Cancer Treatment

Maria C. Figueroa

I t is bad enough to have cancer and have to go through the journey of treatment, but some people also experience financial devastation with this disease. The financial burden of the cost of care can cause a great deal of stress. Many insurance companies don't provide full coverage, and many people have no insurance coverage at all. If you have medical insurance, it is very important for you to know what your insurance company does and doesn't cover.

My first recommendation to patients undergoing cancer treatment is to talk with your health care team about your financial situation as soon as possible. They might have local information or recommendations specific to your situation that can be of assistance. I also recommend inquiring if the cancer center where you are receiving treatment has a patient navigator. Patient navigators are "trained, culturally sensitive health care workers who provide support and guidance throughout the cancer care continuum. They help people 'navigate' through the maze of doctors' offices, clinics, hospitals, outpatient centers, [and] insurance and payment systems. . . ." (http://crchd.cancer.gov/pnp/what-are.html). Nearly all major cancer centers throughout the United States have patient navigators, some of whom are sponsored by the American Cancer Society and have a wealth of information to assist patients with their needs (call 1-800-ACS-2345 to learn if there's a patient navigator program in your area). If you are being treated at a cancer center that doesn't have a patient navigator, ask to speak with a social worker.

The medications used for chemotherapy are usually the most expensive part of cancer treatment. If you have a problem with co-payments or don't have insurance coverage, ask if your social worker or patient navigator can help you access a *medication assistance program*. Many pharmaceutical companies have patient assistance programs that provide support. If such a program is offered, you will be introduced to a person who interviews you and completes an application on your behalf. The application is then submitted to the various drug companies that provide the drugs needed for your treatment. The process takes a few days, so if you are diagnosed with cancer and need this type of assistance, I recommend that you request this service right away.

You might also qualify for assistance from a government program. Federal programs such as Medicare, Medicaid, and Social Security provide medical assistance. These services target people who are disabled or elderly or who have low incomes—so, even if you are not elderly, cancer might result in your being able to qualify as having a disability or having a low income. If you are 62 years of age or older and need education, advocacy, legal assistance, and/or health care, contact the Center for Medicare Advocacy, Inc. by calling 860-456-7790 or visiting www.medicareadvocacy.org.

Medicaid is a state-run health insurance program available to people with limited incomes. You must meet certain requirements to be eligible, including whether your income and your assets and resources (such as bank accounts, property, and things that can be sold for cash) meet certain established criteria. The rules concerning your income level and resources vary from state to state. Special rules apply to people living in nursing homes and disabled children living at home. Your child may be covered by Medicaid even if you are not. If someone else's child lives with you, that child may be eligible based on his or her status, not yours. For more information about Medicaid eligibility, visit the Centers for Medicare and Medicaid Services (CMS) Web site at www.cms.hhs.gov/MedicaidEligibility. Even if you are not sure if you qualify for Medicaid, it's a good idea to apply and let a caseworker in your state evaluate your circumstances.

Many state governments offer additional programs to assist qualified residents with medical expenses. These programs have a lengthy process, so the sooner you submit your paperwork the better. Patient navigators and social workers have information regarding government programs and can assist you with the application process.

Specific Programs That Can Help

U.S. Oncology offers *Oncology Reimbursement Solutions* (ORS) *Patient Assistance Support* (http://www.orsoncology.com/patient_assistance_support.aspx) as a centralized resource to assist practices in helping secure financial support for patients in need. If you lack coverage or are underinsured, the ORS Patient Assistance Support group will work with your practice to acquire the financial support you need through patient assistance programs. Also, many providers will work with patients to schedule monthly payment plans.

CancerCare provides limited financial assistance for pain medication, home care, child care, and transportation for patients with all types of cancers, as well as limited assistance to pay for hormonal and oral chemotherapy, anti-nausea medication, lymphedema supplies, and durable medical equipment for patients with breast cancer. The Cancer-Care Web site (www.cancercare.org) also offers a free resource guide titled *A Helping Hand* that lists national and local resources for cancer services. If you have extensive insurance co-pays, contact the Cancer-Care Co-Payment Assistance Foundation at 866-552-6729, or visit www.cancercarecopay.org.

You can also contact the *Patient Advocate Foundation Co-Pay Relief Program* (866-512-3861; www.copays.org). This organization provides direct co-payment assistance for pharmaceutical products to insured patients who may qualify financially and medically. Please note that funds are limited and the amount of funding available can change. It is best to contact this program right away if you know that you are going to need help.

If you need to travel a long distance for your treatment, contact *Air Charity Network* (previously known as Angel Flight America). This organization provides free flights to people in need of medical treatment. For information about an affiliate in your area, call 877-621-7177 or visit www.aircharitynetwork.org.

The *Health Well Foundation* provides financial assistance to patients with breast cancer, colorectal cancer, and certain lymphomas. This foundation considers a patient's medical, financial, and insurance situation when determining eligibility. You may qualify if your family income is up to four times the federal poverty level. If you qualify, the Health Well Foundation will grant you full or partial assistance for up to 12 months. For more information, visit to www.healthwellfoundation.org.

The *Chronic Disease Fund* offers to pay some out-of-pocket expenses for underinsured patients with breast cancer, colorectal cancer, multiple myeloma, and non-small cell lung cancer. The fund considers income levels by geographic area and the number of household dependents. Visit www.cdfund.org for more information.

Finally, organizations in your community may offer help with transportation, lodging, and home care costs for cancer care. Local chapters of the *American Cancer Society* may provide volunteer drivers to take you to and from physician appointments and treatment. You should also contact your local *United Way* to see if they are able to assist you.

Legal Issues That Can Impact Your Financial Status

It is also important to know your legal rights. A number of laws protect your rights as a patient regarding health insurance and related matters, such as:

* The *Family and Medical Leave Act* (FMLA), which provides eligible employees with up to 12 weeks of unpaid job protected leave per year beyond whatever sick leave you may have accrued at work. It also requires employers to maintain your group health benefits during the leave. For more information, visit www.dol.gov.
* The *Consolidated Omnibus Budget Reconciliation Act* (COBRA) gives workers and their families the right to continue group health insurance benefits for a limited time, usually 18 months, due to loss of job, reduced work hours, or other life events.
* The *Health Insurance Portability and Accountability Act* (HIPAA) prohibits discrimination against employees and their dependents enrolled in group health plans based on their health status.
* The *Americans with Disabilities Act* (ADA) prohibits employment discrimination against qualified individuals with disabilities, including those whose cancer has resulted in disability (http://www.eeoc.gov/facts/cancer.html). As only one example, in 2009, an employer agreed to pay "$125,000 and furnish significant remedial relief to settle a disability discrimination lawsuit filed by the U.S. Equal Employment Opportunity Commission" on behalf of a breast cancer survivor (http://www.eeoc.gov/press/7-22-09.html).

CHAPTER 13

Finding Strength and Celebrating Life

Rose Gordon

Most of my friends and acquaintances who had cancer survived it. Their cancers were caught early and treated—they defeated ovarian cancer, colon cancer, breast cancer, and throat cancer. Treatment has improved greatly, and cancer is no longer the death sentence it used to be. My husband, John, was diagnosed with early stage prostate cancer 11 months ago, received radioactive seed implants, and is doing very well, with no signs of metastasis. John has a positive mental attitude. He goes to the gym six days a week and stays active. My brother Pat was diagnosed four years ago with stage IV small cell lung cancer and was given less than a year to live. He is now cancer free after chemo and radiation.

All of these instances of cancer were life-changing experiences for those who were looking at the possible end of their lives. Did they do things right in their lives? Did they have to make any amends? Was it time to change a few things? Did they have time to clean out a few closets, drawers, and files so no one else would have to? Could they become a better parent, child, sibling, or friend? Could they draw closer to God for strength and comfort during the difficult days of treatment ahead? Yes, many reported life-changing experiences, and most will say cancer has made them better people.

"Cancer has been a blessing in my life," my best friend, Jan, explained as we agonized over her recent news that cancer had returned. "As hard as it is for people to understand, and in spite of the pain and suffering I have had to endure these past 12 years," she continued, "it has made me a better person." After exhausting every possibility for a cure, including surgeries, radiation, meditation, prayer and faith healing, counseling, vitamins, and exercise, she came to realize that sometimes the answer for healing is "no." It crossed her mind that stress may play a role in developing cancer.

Jan was a nurse and continued working between and through her treatments until it became too difficult physically. As much as she loved life, her husband, her home and family, travel, and me, she knew that life was temporal and we all get one crack at it, yet life goes on after we leave this realm. She loved each moment, each day, and lived them to the fullest; Jan was a "YES, LET'S!" kind of person with a ready laugh and a great sense of humor. Once I asked Jan to write a recommendation for me for a job that I really wanted. Several days later she handed me a business envelope; I opened the letter carefully so as not to crinkle it before I presented my glowing recommendation to my future employer. I read:

> Rose is the type of friend that comes along only once or twice in a lifetime. We have shared experiences only a lifetime of friendship can endure. We have laughed till we cried and cried till we laughed. We played in the Florida sun, watched Evel Knievel jump 15 buses in Ohio; we slept in tents in the middle of forests and cooked over open campfires. We stayed in the most posh hotels in the big metropolitan cities and dined in the finest of restaurants. We prayed together at night in a hospital room in Indianapolis. We've both raised lovely daughters who are friends. Rose and I have shared being single and we shared our wedding days. Through the happiest moments and the darkest of hours we have stood by each other's side. We've walked through woods, on the beaches, in the malls and down church aisles. We drank a few beers and smoked a few joints (*but never inhaled*) and partied until the break of dawn. We have brought each other souvenir magnets from our individual travels all over the world. She and I have enjoyed life, and the best part is, we have both been "born again," so I know we'll have each other's friendship for all eternity. Through thick and thin. Love, Jan

It was her letter *to me*—to always remember our fun times. Then she handed me the real recommendation for my future employer, rather dry and boring; she kept it politically correct while focusing on my business attributes. I got the job.

Jan did not give up the fight, but rather had come to the quiet acceptance of her impending transition. She grew weary of the battle and just wanted to think about and do other things besides fight cancer. She also knew that sometimes the answer to our prayer is not always what we want it to be. She had a strong faith and knew one way or another that this, too, would pass. She loved rainbows—they were a promise from God, the Bible says, and always a big event when one appeared in the sky after a rainstorm. She collected them in various forms and related the cancer to a big storm she was caught up in while she waited for the rainbow.

Jan wasn't afraid of dying, she just didn't like the thought of the actual process of it. She said that if God had given her an option on how she wanted to leave this world, she still would have chosen cancer and not a sudden heart attack or car accident. This disease, she said, gave her time to get her house in order and say the things that needed to be said and mend relationships that needed mending and get her daughter through college.

One day I stopped to see Jan while she was recovering from another round of chemo. She had stopped mid-treatment, stating she had had enough and was not going to be put through any more of it. I sat on the floor and cried at her knees, knowing she had made her decision and she was fine with it. I bemoaned the fact that it was so difficult for me to lose my best friend and attempted to put into words everything I felt in my heart. She interrupted my babble and told me then that she and I had enjoyed a wonderful 20-year friendship, that few do, and that over those years we had said it all and had done so many things that other people only talk about. We both started laughing hysterically when she said, "I don't believe in trying to cram a whole lifetime into the last five minutes."

She was right. That made me feel better, but I continued wailing at the foot of her chair at the unfairness of it all and why a good person like her had to go through all of this suffering and not some murderer or rapist who only burdened society with their evil deeds. I certainly had not come to that point where she was, the point of quiet understanding. As I wiped my tears, she patted my head while calmly reassuring me that I would be okay. There she was, consoling *me*; she had a way of always turning things around. She told me when she got to heaven she was going to run with the angels, but she wouldn't forget me. Then we made a pact. I told her if she were to make it there before me (we always reasoned that nothing was preventing me from dying before her in an accident or something), that if there was any way possible that God would allow her to let me know she made it in, she would. She emphatically said, "If there is *any* way at all for me to let you know, I will." I promised to do the same.

The next day I had to leave for a three-day business trip. I hated to leave while she was steadily losing ground, but the trip was a necessity. While on the road, I would look for a new rainbow gift for her—a picture, magnet, or music box, anything with a rainbow to bring her a flicker of hope and a smile. I was unable to find time to shop for a gift and then had a four-hour trip home after the trade show. I called to see how she was doing. Her husband, Rey, said she was not doing well. While driving home, I was hit by the senselessness of her struggle. I began praying, asking God *why* she had not been healed, *why* he had not answered her prayers, *why* all the suffering, and *why* not the guy who just killed all those people? I felt a growing anger in my heart at God for not healing her as He did Job.

As I drove, I could see the storm clouds brewing in the distance and knew I was heading right into a big one. It began to rain. I turned off the highway onto a rural road for the next two- hour stretch home. My soul was filled with the anguish of Jan's ordeal with cancer, and rage began overflowing inside me. I began lashing out at God, demanding an answer to her suffering. The sky darkened as my own tornado welled up inside me. The wind picked up and rain began pelting my van. I was alone with God and began crying out in my pent-up grief, ranting and raving out loud like a mad woman as the tears flooded my face. The torrential rain hammered down and the wind buffeted my van to and fro, swaying it down the road. The trees were bending back and forth in a riveting dance with the wind. My hands tightly gripped the steering wheel as two frontal systems collided; the lightning and thunder cracking and flashing around me and my own voice battling back in defiance.

It felt as if I were in a wrestling match with God, but it was no contest. I felt defeated by the force of nature and the force of His might. Weakened and emotionally spent from fighting against the Power of the universe, I knew I had to let go and accept the inevitable. This was the circle of life, and I knew that—I was selfishly decrying my own loss. God certainly did not have to answer to me, but I still wanted a response. Soon the storm subsided along with my tears. It was getting lighter outside, and the rain was now a fine sprinkle. As I drove, arched against a blue sky over a golden cornfield was the most magnificent double rainbow! Jan's rainbow!

It was nothing short of amazing. I marveled at the spectacle before me and the intensity of color. In an undeniable voice of great authority and power, the Lord spoke to my heart. He spoke with distinct clarity and conviction with words I'll never forget: "I have *not* forgotten Jan!" I knew who had spoken and felt totally penitent and humbled. A sense of peace washed over me, and my tears of anger turned into tears of joy as I sat in amazement at the brilliant rainbow before me—His promise. The scripture came to me: "I set My rainbow in the cloud, and it shall be for the sign of the covenant between Me and the earth" (Genesis 9:13). He heard Jan's prayers, and He heard mine. I was renewed of spirit and knew right then that there was more to life than cancer could ever take away. I rushed home to phone Jan and tell her about what had just happened. I told her that the Lord had revealed to me His promise and that He had heard her prayers and she had not been forgotten. She thanked me for telling her about the rainbow and then said, "I love you, now I have to go." Those were her last words to me. I was there the next day when she made the transition, and I was at peace knowing that she, too, was at peace. Her spirit lives on.

Jan had asked me to give her eulogy, and her husband had me pick out her funeral card. I found the perfect card with her favorite flower, the iris, on it and chose this verse—The Prayer of St. Francis of Assisi:

> Lord, make me an instrument of your peace. Where there is hatred, let me sow love. Where there is injury, pardon. Where there is doubt, faith. Where there is despair, hope. Where there is darkness, light and where there is sadness, joy. O Divine Master, grant that I may not so much seek to be consoled as to console; to be understood as to understand; to be loved as to love. For it is in giving that we receive; it is pardoning that we are pardoned; and it is in dying that we are born to eternal life.

It was October, so I ordered mums from the local farmer's market for the service. My order was for 10 potted plants, with the agreement that I would pick them up on my way to the chapel for the service. When I arrived at the farmer's market, the farmer from whom I had ordered the mums had not arrived! I became panicky, not knowing what to do, not having any flowers for Jan, and the service was to start in two hours.

Frantically I prayed, "What shall I do, Lord? *I need the mums!*" My husband and I tore around the market hoping to find something—the market was swarming with people, and what happened next was nothing short of miraculous. When we got to the other end of the market, a big truck was just pulling up, loaded with, of all things, unbelievably huge mums! I flagged down the farmer, telling him I needed 10 mums right away! They were *three times* the size of the mums that I had ordered and were *half* the cost! The farmer seemed very happy to oblige this crazy lady who was demanding so many before he even had a chance to unload them. As he hurried to unload the most colorful mums, he commented that his day had started off wrong, but it seemed to be turning around for him now. I told him that he was an answer to my prayer!

I thanked the Lord profusely as we put the pots of mums into the back of our SUV. On the way to the chapel, we stopped at the grocery store for floral paper and ribbon. We wrapped the pots of mums in pretty paper and bows, arriving at the service in plenty of time. Jan's brothers helped unload the mums to the oohs and ahhs of her elderly aunts, who were tickled to learn that each would be taking a mum home with her. The arrangement formed a beautiful rainbow behind the memorial table. I know Jan was smiling and shaking her head.

Over a year later, I had a dream. Jan appeared to me in my dream, smiling and glowing with radiant health and youthfulness. She had baby's breath in her hair, as she did on her wedding day, and she was wearing soft, flowing, cream-colored cotton apparel. I was startled and yet excited to see her. "JAN!" There were so many things I wanted to say and ask her, and there were so many questions and so much catching up that I wanted to do. My mind was whirling, but after exclaiming her name, nothing else would come out. My mouth moved, trying to form words. As hard as I tried to speak, I was mute.

Tears were rolling down my cheeks—joy at being able to see her again. Jan continued smiling at me, seemingly amused at my predicament, yet somehow *knowing*. Finally, I blurted out, "Are you in heaven?!" She answered, "Yes," and then she was gone. I woke up, crying, and saw that it was four o'clock in the morning. I knew I had had a visitation from Jan. God often used dreams in the Bible to reveal great things—the birth of Jesus, for one—and Jan, keeping true to her word, came back in a dream to let me know she had made it to heaven. I had forgotten our pact, figuring there was not a way.

How clever for Jan to use a dream rather than some mysterious sign that I always would have wondered about! Neither of us believed in ghosts or apparitions, which are never of God. I figured she worked it out with Him that she would appear in my dream, a mode He does use, and, providing I asked the right question, she would be given one word to answer. He silenced my lips until I found the right question.

Jan's illness was my introduction to cancer and a major loss of someone I dearly loved. There is a Power greater than ourselves that surrounds and comforts us through the dark moments when we feel alone and depleted of strength, understanding, and faith. There were many instances when I felt His presence. Events with Jan would help prepare me for later trials in my life. We are all given challenges in life, and with each one there are learning experiences. We develop new strengths to endure future challenges. Unfortunately, we are not always aware of seeming coincidences—the sighting of rainbows, huge mums replacing those ordered. Not happenstance at all, but rather in the moment of great anguish, He tapped me on the shoulder and said, "Look."

CHAPTER 14

Finding Untapped Resources and Learning New Skills through Professional Counseling

Joyce A. DeVoss

Once the diagnosis of cancer is made, the person with cancer and his or her loved ones are faced with many challenges that they may have never before had to address and for which they feel totally unprepared. One of their first challenges is accepting the diagnosis. Cancer is typically perceived as a life-threatening diagnosis that is not taken lightly. Each family member may have a uniquely individual way of coping. Some might cope by openly becoming emotional. Others might repress their feelings so as not to upset the cancer patient or themselves. Some family members might engage in unhealthy activities such as substance abuse in an attempt to cope with the diagnosis. By engaging a professional counselor soon after the cancer diagnosis, family members can avoid self-destructive methods of coping and receive encouragement for the use of healthy coping approaches. A counselor also can assist family members in developing new skills and resiliency for coping not only with the current challenges but also with those that lie ahead.

Counselor as Family Care Team Member

A professionally trained counselor can serve as an important member of a multidisciplinary care team of the cancer patient and his or her family. Professional counselors have expertise in crisis management and skills for helping clients sort out issues and develop perspective on their circumstances. A counselor who has specialized training in helping families impacted by cancer can help his or her clients manage a range of common and predictable emotions that may be quite disturbing for the family dealing with cancer. A counselor can also serve as a consultant to the other professionals involved with the cancer patient and his or her family, as well as an advocate for the patient and family. The professional counselor can make a significant contribution to the care and well-being of the cancer patient and family.

Counselors know how to help families tap into their strengths, as well as look for opportunities within what may appear, at first glance, to be a completely dismal situation. In addition, they can help family members to anticipate and prepare for future events, such as various cancer treatments that might put additional demands on the resources of the cancer patient's family.

The cancer patient and family members may experience worry and anxiety about the possible death of the patient. Children in the family may experience fear, separation anxiety, somatic complaints, sleep and appetite changes, and inhibition in school (see chapter 4). Adult family members may experience a range of cognitive, emotional, and somatic symptoms that impact their daily functioning at home, at work, and in social settings. Over time, symptoms associated with worry and anxiety take a toll on the resiliency of the human spirit. A counselor can help family members to sort out realistic versus unrealistic fears. If the cancer patient is told by the doctor that he or she is dying, the counselor can help the family to explore strategies to best take advantage of the time they have left with their loved one and at the same time address some anticipatory grief issues.

Additional stressors on the family can heighten the impact of cancer in a family member on the entire family system—for instance, financial stress, homelessness, other psychological or medical problems, substance abuse, recent deaths or other losses, legal problems, or other stressors. Family members can learn how to address daily issues associated with having a cancer patient in the family. There may be a dramatic change in priorities directly associated with the impact of cancer. Frequently, there is a major impact upon the finances of the family. Additionally, family members typically experience increased demands on their time for caretaking tasks associated with the cancer patient. There may be a noticeable change in the types of activities in which the family engages. For example, very active families might change the types of activities the family members do together to those that are less physically demanding in order to include the cancer patient.

Any one or combinations of these or other challenges can create a crisis for one or more family members, requiring a new set of coping skills that are beyond those adequate for most stresses of daily living. When family members encounter stress beyond their capability to cope and the extended family has reached their limits as a support network, struggling family members, also considered co-survivors of cancer, are likely to benefit from professional assistance. For some individuals, the news of a cancer diagnosis for a loved one leads to a downward spiraling series of experiences that might include worry, anxiety, and other emotional problems, sleep problems, appetite problems, work or school performance inhibition, impaired social relationships, questioning of faith, and other symptoms. For those with preexisting emotional disorders, the news of the cancer diagnosis within the family can exacerbate their emotional difficulties and develop into a crisis.

Cancer patients and their loved ones need not wait until they experience a crisis before they contact a counselor. They can engage in counseling on an individual or family basis at any point in the process of coping with cancer. A proactive approach to the impact of cancer involves the inclusion of a professional counselor as part of the care plan for cancer patients and their families. Early involvement of a family impacted by cancer with a professional counselor provides a resource and outlet for the cancer patient and co-survivors when they are vulnerable, at risk, and likely to benefit from what a counselor has to offer.

Changing Family Roles

A professional counselor can help a cancer patient's family to anticipate changing family roles. When cancer comes to a family, the family members are confronted with the necessity for redistributed, new, and never-planned-for roles, including "cancer patient" and "caregivers." Caregiving may address the needs of the cancer patient or another family member—for instance, a young child's or elderly family member's needs that were previously met by the cancer patient. If the cancer patient was a "breadwinner" in the family and has to quit or take an extended leave from his or her job, another family member might have to find work or increase work hours in order to make up for lost income.

Household chores may be redistributed in a family facing cancer, possibly causing resentment and interference with other activities and preferred ways of spending time. With the help of counseling, a family can minimize some of the negative consequences of changing family roles by allowing family members to express their feelings, offer support for one another, and incorporate a democratic process with flexibility as they decide how to share the load.

Caregiver's Fatigue

A counselor can be helpful to the caregivers of the cancer patient by alerting them to the potential for caregiver's fatigue and ways for preventing it. Care of the cancer patient can lead caretakers to experience extreme fatigue from the demands of that role added to the day-to-day demands of the other roles the caregivers fulfill. Caregivers often take on their roles without considering the physical, psychological, and other costs of caregiving because there may be no other choice. They may not be aware of risks for caregiver fatigue until they actually experience physical and emotional signs of the impact on their well-being, such as sleep and appetite problems, headaches, stomachaches, anxiety, depression, irritability, emotionality, exhaustion, etc. The professional counselor can assist caregivers in planning good self-care, including healthy diet, regular exercise, effective use of a social support system, arranging for respite on a regular basis, and developing awareness of early signs of caregiver's fatigue.

Cultural and Spiritual Issues

Professional counselors can support families facing cancer in one of their members by encouraging them to include in their support system (if they haven't already) trusted members of the extended family or designated helpers within the family's cultural and/or spiritual community, such as *curanderos*, medicine men or women, priests, rabbis, and ministers, who offer additional sources of support and assist in the family's time of need. Families who have such supports are likely to experience a greater sense of hope and calmness in the midst of the burdens created on their family system by cancer. Prayer and religious rituals can provide a sense of meaning and hope and an effective outlet for family members as they deal with their own sense of helplessness in the face of cancer. The professional counselor can offer family members respect and flexibility in incorporating their cultural and spiritual beliefs into their treatment in order to accommodate their personal needs over the course of the family's challenges with cancer.

Reactions of Others

A professional counselor can help a family with a cancer patient face the decision of what and when to tell others and how much information to share. Sometimes, family members may experience shame or embarrassment about the cancer diagnosis. The patient or family members may feel guilty for not changing unhealthy lifestyle choices such as smoking, consuming alcohol and/or other substances, overeating, and lack of exercise. Family members may wish that they had done more to influence the cancer patient to change his or her unhealthy habits. They may also be concerned that they themselves will eventually be diagnosed with cancer. The counselor can assist family members in working through their feelings and reservations about telling others about the cancer diagnosis and help them to anticipate the reactions and questions they may encounter.

Talking to Children

The family might decide to seek out a counselor who has expertise in helping children deal with cancer in the family (see chapter 4). A counselor can help with telling children about the cancer and help them learn to cope as well as they can with the situation. Sometimes children are overlooked or intentionally not told about a cancer diagnosis in the family. Children in this type of situation often sense that something is wrong in the family and become confused when what they observe and sense does not match with what they are told. This may create a great deal of stress for the children. It is helpful for children to have a professional with whom they can share their feelings and concerns—to be able to ask questions and get answers that are honest and developmentally appropriate. In addition, it is helpful for the children's therapist to meet with the adults in the family to share tips with them on how to help their children cope.

When a Child Is the Cancer Patient

A child cancer patient needs to have his or her psychological needs assessed and a plan developed to meet those needs. The plan is likely to include counseling for the child with a specialist who treats children with medical issues such as cancer. The counselor is part of the child's professional care team and can serve as an individual counselor to the child, family counselor for the parents and siblings, and consultant to the other professionals involved in the child's treatment. In the counselor's work with the individual child, he or she may use psychoeducational approaches, play therapy, art therapy, bibliotherapy, and other child-friendly approaches designed to assist children in expressing feelings and concerns and working through them. The counselor is likely to work with other professionals involved with the child and family. For example, the child's educational needs should be assessed by an educational specialist and a plan developed and implemented to meet those needs (see chapter 3). The counselor can offer the educational team insight into the child's motivation for learning and suggest strategies that might be most effective in promoting the child's academic success.

The Long Haul

If cancer becomes a chronic illness or disability in a family member, coping over a long period of time may involve numerous and various types of treatments over periods of months to years and corresponding adjustments within family roles and routines. These ongoing adjustments require that families tap into previously developed resiliency skills or acquire new ones. These are skills that increase a person's ability to recover from adversity and to learn from the experience so that the person can successfully adapt while dealing with stressors in life. A professional counselor can help the cancer survivor and family reframe the cancer as a challenge rather than a defeat.

The family can be encouraged to persist through setbacks and problems and support one another in circumstances over which they may have little or no control. Families can learn to invest their energy in focusing on where they can make a difference. The family can be urged to thoroughly enjoy times when the cancer survivor goes into remission, not allowing fears of recurrence to interfere with living fully.

A counselor is likely to advise the family to advocate for the cancer survivor and for themselves and to be proactive in addressing problems as they arise rather than being passive and allowing small problems to transform into crises. The counselor may emphasize the development of unused or underused resources within the family, building a larger and stronger support system wherein members of the family feel comfortable asking for help. Family members can be reminded by the counselor to engage regularly in relaxing and fun activities that provide joy for them. Furthermore, the counselor can promote a healthy sense of humor in the face of the stress caused for the family by cancer. Sometimes, families need permission of a professional to enjoy themselves despite the burdens caused by cancer in a loved one.

Resources

The professional counselor can point out additional resources for the family, including informational Web sites, telephone numbers, and online and face-to-face support groups. Support services can be identified by focus: on the patient, family members, cancer type, and geographical location. Online support groups and services are provided at medical clinics, hospitals, mental health agencies, churches, and other organizations. A co-payment assistance foundation exists for cancer patients. For instance, cancer patients and their family members can access these resources and cancer education materials by visiting www.cancercare.org, calling 1-800-813-HOPE, or e-mailing info@cancercare.org.

Professional Counselor as Broker of Unused Opportunities

The diagnosis of cancer in a family member is clearly a challenging life event for both the cancer patient and family members. A professional counselor engaged with the family can assist the family in finding "unused opportunities" within these life circumstances. For instance, the counselor can engage the family members in a process that may enable them to become closer as they work together to support their loved one and each other. In addition, the counselor can help family members learn more about cancer and to become more proactive in making their own lifestyle changes to reduce their cancer risk. Furthermore, the counselor can assist family members in reflecting on their lives, recognizing what is most important to them, and realigning their goals for a more meaningful life experience.

PART 3

LIVING BEYOND CANCER

CHAPTER 15

When Cancer Came Home: Memories of My Mother, Directions for My Life

Rebecca Paradies

Cancer came home while I wasn't looking. It snuck in through the back door like an unwanted guest, leaving its dirty footprints all over my life. My emotions had nowhere to go, so they often came out sideways, unleashed on some unexpected victim. I would enter into a new relationship and somewhere in the back of my mind expect that that person too would die too soon. Cancer stole my mother and left me with questions of how to be. I grew up with the shadow of cancer around every corner. I wasn't a small child, but I was not yet fully formed as an adult. My mother was just able to see that I would be okay in life and that possibly I would become a contributing adult in society. Her last note to me, as cancer left her unable to speak, asked if I had graduated from college. I lied and shook my head yes.

Cancer came home and acted like a backseat driver in everything I did. I have recently turned the age my mother was when she died after a two-year struggle with non-Hodgkin's lymphoma. While I rejoiced at this milestone, I am keenly aware of how scared she must have been. I live daily with the possibility that life could be taken away. In a sense, cancer has given me a right to live more fully, to follow my passion, to experience this life the best way I can, and to honor my mother by attempting to live a more compassionate life.

Upon my mother's death, I was the logical choice among siblings to move back home. Having been gone for eight years, I would help my father adjust to his new life as a widower. He was used to me not being there; I was not used to viewing my father in a new light—someone other than the distant intermittent raging authoritarian. We had a lot of mending to do. We learned how to cook basic foods, mastered the washing machine, and mostly learned how to navigate through memories in the house that had previously held so much pain. I didn't stay long, but long enough for my father to be able to cook several meals, separate the lights from the darks, and begin to think of a new way of being in the world. I, in turn, gained a new relationship with my father. We became very close, and he would refer to me not only as his daughter, but as his friend.

When there is a life transition such as a loss in a family, often our roles shift. In this transition, I became an adult and a caregiver. My father became dependent on me—our roles reversed for the first time. I remember the exact moment it happened; I was making the bed for my aunty Jean, my mother's older sister, who stayed with us after the funeral. The awareness of my new position sunk in so deeply that I was momentarily crippled by the sheer weight of the responsibility. I made the bed with a new intention, placed fresh flowers on the nightstand, and looked for a reasonably new towel with matching washcloth.

As I was cleaning the bathroom, the one my mother used, I noticed on the back of the toilet my mother's black reading glasses, waiting for the next romance novel to be read. I picked them up almost in reverence as some sacred object, and put them on, hoping to see what she might have seen in the mirror just a few weeks before. Did she know she was dying? Did she leave a note telling me how proud she was of me? Did she love enough? I placed them back where I had found them, hoping the rightful owner would return. I cried and closed the door, knowing that was not to be. I began to look for something else to straighten.

The next 20 years were filled with the usual experiences: marriage, birth of a beautiful child, everyday challenges, and eventually a painful divorce. Where was my mother? I needed her wisdom, guidance, and strength. I am certain that if my mother had not died, I surely would have made a much better marriage choice. At least I hope to think I would have listened. During these difficult times of divorce, when I would feel particularly helpless and vulnerable, I could feel her presence sitting beside me, just as she had done when I was a child. I began to call on her spirit often and would eventually refer to my mother as my "invisible means of support." I would write to her of my life and of her granddaughter, who was growing into a spirited child and teenager, much as I had been.

Often I would find myself looking down at my own hands and see hers, whether driving her 1979 diesel Mercedes I inherited, or looking through her recipe box of carefully hand-written recipes on index cards. I would run my fingers along the lines and trace her loopy Os and dramatically crossed Ts. This box was often a favorite toy of my daughter—her granddaughter—the one she never got to meet. Julia would organize the contents as only a three-year-old could do. Recipes like Fruit Mallo Dip, consisting primarily of marshmallow and mayonnaise, or perhaps Apple Sauce Salad, which included a package of lemon Jell-O and candy. Needless to say, she was not the best of cooks. However, her dishes were always creative, if not sometimes a mystery. I became a vegetarian in my teens while questioning her ingredients; I must have frustrated her to no end.

I finally grew into the woman I am today, complete with my own set of odd recipes, eccentricities, and wonderment of how she was able to raise three children. My mother would single-handedly cart us off in various directions, give us every opportunity for success, love without judgment, and place curious food on the table every evening. At the time of her diagnosis and two years of treatment, I lived 100 miles away. I was not able to go to, nor did she want to involve me in, her chemotherapy sessions. My mother was a private woman, and up until her death, no one knew how sick she was; this was her way of dealing with cancer. I imagine it was her and my father's decision together how to travel that most difficult road.

My mother's cancer journey helped influence my decision to attend graduate school. I became an expressive arts therapist. My first internship was with breast cancer survivors. I would arrive to group equipped with painting materials, a variety of musical instruments, costumes, and expectations. I would help these women proceed through their disease with creative expression. I quickly realized my plan was not to go as prescribed. These women were used to being told what to do, when to show up for treatment, what food to avoid for nausea, and so on. To a certain extent, their disease dictated their lives. The expressive arts group was a place for them to be able to reclaim some control; I went along for the ride. I provided the tools and held the space for creativity and expression.

Whatever I thought I was bringing to them, I quickly realized that they brought much more to me. I learned how to let go of my expectations, agendas, and preconceived notions; I learned how to listen. The women taught me humor in the face of a crisis, compassion, and how to sit with uncomfortable emotions. Through these women, I was able to gain an insight into my mother's cancer experience and was more fully able to connect with her.

Today, I am an expressive arts therapist working on a locked psychiatric unit with adults who are unable to fully function in the outside world. I try to bring to my work all of the wisdom and lessons learned from the cancer survivor groups that I was privileged to be a part of, from my father, who has long passed, and from the memory and strength of my mother. I continue to write and paint and often feel the spirit of my mother enter into my work and reside between the lines of poetry I write. I feel her gentleness when I attempt to console my now-grown daughter and her strength as I move into the second half of my life. Cancer came home and settled in long ago, and I have learned to make peace with it and give it acknowledgement for its unexpected gifts. With that said, however, I would gladly prefer to have my mother here with me, holding hands and sharing recipes.

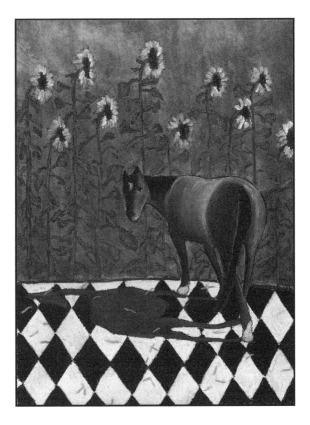

Cutter, by Rebecca Paradies.

CHAPTER 16

Finding Your Own Way: Living with Chronic Illness or a Shade of Gray

Anne Mallett

Tears stung my eyes as I forcefully clicked off my phone. Having a doctor decline my case is nothing out of the ordinary for me, but this one hit a new low. After I had spent more than an hour in the office, this particular doctor had yelled at my seven-year-old son for rocking back and forth in his chair. My son had seen this doctor grab my neck so forcefully that I nearly fell off the table. I had to explain to my son that the doctor didn't mean to throw my medical records at me when he stated he felt uncomfortable taking my case and would have to ponder the request further. I knew this doctor's rejection was coming from a mile away. I just wish I hadn't brought my son along as a witness. I only did it because the doctor's office was an hour's drive to the city, and afterward I wanted to take my son to the zoo.

My plight into the medical world started on March 5, 2003. I woke up and instantly knew something was terribly wrong. My mouth had enormous ulcers in it; I felt nauseated. As days went on, I became weak, feverish, and struggled with night chills. I saw doctor after doctor, to no avail. Each doctor had his or her own theory as to what was causing my decline. I would faithfully accept the diagnosis and take prescribed medication in hopes of relief. Nothing was working. I then ended up with an infectious disease control doctor who was highly regarded in the medical community. I thought that surely he would save the day.

After eight days in the hospital, I became frightened that he would never let me out, so I asked for a second opinion. Wow, did that bruise his ego and cause him to write malicious lies in my medical records. He declined to give me the CT scan that I requested, wrote that I could be self-inducing my symptoms, and reported that I had Obsessive-Compulsive Disorder. At that point, I didn't even care what he wrote in my chart as long as I could leave the hospital. Feeling weary, I just wanted to go back home to care for my family.

After several months and doctors from every medical specialty, I started to lose hope. I began to think, "Maybe that infectious disease doctor was right and I'm just losing my mind." I knew in my heart that it couldn't be true. As a student getting ready to graduate with her Master of Social Work degree, I knew enough about mental health to know that I couldn't possibly just be imagining my symptoms. They were too real. The effects were too devastating: my hair falling out, my fatigue, my skin breaking out into a rash, my mouth so infected with ulcers, thrush, and the bacteria seeping from my tonsils couldn't possibly just be a figment of my imagination. I feverishly began to read books on Holocaust survivors as my only source of strength and perspective.

I kept having this deep sense that I was going to die, and my body's breakdown each day was confirming my worst fears. I decided I would continue to persevere and see as many doctors as possible until one would listen to me and validate my concerns. One day in June 2003, I decided to see a gastroenterologist. He was a kind man who very thoughtfully listened to the laundry list of symptoms that I was suffering from at the time. This doctor decided to do what no other doctor up to that point had considered doing—he decided to give me a basic physical examination.

As he checked my body over, I recall thinking how elementary his approach was and began to doubt that this man knew what he was doing. When he got to my right abdominal wall, he gently pushed down and then looked up at me, concerned. With resignation, he stated that I had a mass near my kidney and that I would benefit from a CT scan. "Oh, really?" I said as I reflected on how I was denied the opportunity to have one through the infectious disease control doctor when I was in the hospital months earlier.

When I received my CT scan, we discovered that I had a 7 cm mass on my right kidney and two 11 cm enlarged lymph nodes in my abdominal wall next to it. Surgery to remove the mass and enlarged lymph nodes was immediately scheduled for four days later. During the surgery, they not only removed the mass and enlarged lymph nodes, but they also did biopsies of my mouth to try and discover the cause of my severe oral concerns. The results were inconclusive for lymphoma, and I received mixed results from the oral biopsies. I didn't really have a solid diagnosis, but the prognosis for me was supposed to be good with the removal of the mass and lymph nodes.

Although I felt slightly better for a few weeks after my surgery, it really wasn't sustaining. I completed my graduate degree and obtained a part-time job as a therapist in hopes that things would turn around regarding my symptoms. I figured my body just needed more time to heal. Unfortunately, I started to get much worse and discovered eight months later that I had another mass on my right kidney measuring 5 cm wide, as well as enlarged lymph nodes throughout my right abdominal side. To top it off, my oral issues continued to become exacerbated to the point that I was nearly unable to speak.

By this time, I decided that I didn't care how much it was going to cost me—I was going to seek the best medical care in the country. I went to a top five medical center, where they removed the mass, removed all the lymph nodes on my right abdominal wall, and cauterized the lesions in my mouth. They also gave me a diagnosis. They reported to me that I had Paraneoplastic Pemphigus with Castleman's Disease and Lymphadenopathy. I ended up flying to another top five medical center to have to my diagnosis confirmed by the world's leading expert.

The medical community saw my illness as part canceresque and part autoimmune. The doctors debate the differences of Castleman's Disease—some say it's cancer and others say it's a shade of gray between benign masses and a precursor to cancer. The doctors also debate the autoimmune piece of my illness, with some saying it's a form of my body attacking itself and others saying that since they can't always detect through tests when and where the attacks are occurring, they can't treat it. As doctors debate amongst themselves about my case, I end up not getting care from anyone. It can be quite discouraging, to say the least.

With Paraneoplastic Pemphigus, the odds of survival are typically less than 10%. If it's found in your lungs or gastrointestinal tract, the odds of survival decrease significantly. And, yes, it was in my GI tract. My only saving grace was that with Castleman's Disease you are more likely to survive if it's caught in time. Between the two medical centers, I felt as if I had a good team and a plan for my future. My health started to improve, and hopes of long-term survival were starting to come to fruition. The only thing that was difficult was the knowledge that so few people are ever given the diagnosis. And the ones who do receive it rarely live. So to survive is very much like uncharted territory. Had I not persevered so quickly and persistently, I would have died.

In the past, most people with the illness were diagnosed just before they died or after an autopsy. More doctors are starting to be aware of this rare illness. The leading expert on my illness advised me that at that time only 26 other cases of it in the world had been diagnosed where the individuals were still alive. I'm thankful to have been so persistent in listening to my inner voice and fighting ahead. Otherwise, my son would have missed out on the opportunity to enjoy his mother.

I am pleased to have survived my illness. However, I continue to have lingering side effects that no one in the medical community knows how to treat. I never realized how little doctors knew until my illness struck. Now I struggle with autoimmune issues that no one knows how to diagnose or treat. An oncologist tells me to see a rheumatologist, as I do not have cancer at this time. And a rheumatologist tells me that my case is better handled by the oncology field. So in the end, I don't receive care from either field and instead continue to suffer from my symptoms.

When most doctors discover that I've had Castleman's Disease, they automatically presume I have HIV. There are two types of Castleman's Disease, both very rare. The majority of people who have Castleman's Disease fall into the category that I have, which is called *Unicentric*, and do not have HIV. Even those that fall into the other category, titled *Multicentric*, don't necessarily have HIV, but doctors aren't always aware of that. I feel as if I have to educate each new doctor so that I don't have to repeatedly go through unnecessary testing for HIV each time. It seems silly nowadays, but it appears to me as though most doctors still don't want to treat individuals with an HIV diagnosis.

I've read that there are over 80 different types of autoimmune disorders and that up to 75% of those affected by them are women in their child-bearing years. Autoimmune disorders are also thought to be one of the top 10 leading causes of death in women. Commonly, a woman will have to go through 20, 30, sometimes even 40 different doctors just to have someone take her concerns seriously and find a diagnosis. Doctors typically do not want to take on autoimmune disorder cases unless they are the common ones such as diabetes or arthritis. That leaves victims of the other 78-plus autoimmune disorders out on their own with no one willing to provide them care. Autoimmune disorders are also considered to be too much of a shade a gray that doctors don't know how to treat. Doctors prefer that patients have a clear, scientifically proven diagnosis so they can refer to the copious amounts of research and proven treatments for it. When you are dealing with autoimmune disorders, treatment knowledge is still in its infancy. Doctors become nervous about what road to take, leading them to feel vulnerable to mistakes and possible liabilities issues.

I'm looking forward to the day when technology is available to discover and treat autoimmune disorders. A hundred years ago, we did not have most of the knowledge and technology we do now to treat illnesses such as cancer or diabetes. Now, we have amazing tools to help doctors pursue and confirm a diagnosis. Unfortunately, the tools for detecting and treating autoimmune disorders remain mostly elusive at this time. Blood tests can sometimes be helpful, but it's not a sure bet. And the treatment of autoimmune disorders is usually a round of corticosteroids that can be considered dangerous.

I've had doctors prefer to prescribe me powerfully addictive narcotics such as Oxycontin and Vicodin over the non-narcotic corticosteroid prednisone. The narcotics do not take away my pain, but the corticosteroids do. I sometimes feel like a dope fiend when I go from doctor to doctor begging them to give me just a small dose of prednisone to take the edge off the pain. To prolong the time I can be on corticosteroids, I've been known to cut my tiny pills in half and lick the dust clean just to get every spare speck possible into my body. It's a shame, really. But what can you do? The alternative is far worse, and my ability to function is drastically reduced.

Working a full-time job, running my private practice as a therapist, attending to childrearing responsibilities, participating in family functions, volunteering for two organizations within the community, and completing household maintenance doesn't factor into my body's need for rest and recovery. It's just not an option for me. So if I have to swallow my pride and humble myself before doctors who sometimes abuse their power, I will do it if it means I can score a month's supply of the medication my body desperately needs.

I don't want anyone to get the wrong idea. I do stand up for myself, and I have come a long way. If I had listened to the infectious disease control doctor, I would have died. I've learned to trust my own instincts instead of blindly taking what a doctor says as golden. I encourage women to advocate for themselves and continue to seek treatment in the face of doctors who dismiss their concerns or decline to treat them. For me, it's now about a balance. I do what needs to be done when it needs doing. I continue to seek out expert treatment from top medical centers, but even the doctors there can acknowledge that they don't know everything.

I've discovered that we are all human and imperfect. Finding doctors who haven't lost their compassion for their patients is probably the most central component to obtaining quality care. It's also vitally important to surround yourself with supportive family, friends, and community resources. Countless times I have needed to rely on my in-laws to care for my son while I was at doctor appointment or in the hospital. On more than one occasion, I have enlisted the presence of my best friend to help advocate for me during sessions with my doctors. I have benefitted from the support of my spouse, who has helped me maintain a sense of humor through the worst of times. I've learned to put the trauma of poorly behaved doctors aside to enjoy the time I have been given with my son. I have felt at peace within myself when surrounded by a community of people who support my faith in Judaism. Whatever you can do to help yourself physically, emotionally, and spiritually through this process will enhance your quality of life and present a greater opportunity for keeping your health stable.

Chronic illness has changed the course of my life. I can manage it, but the future just holds more questions than answers. I would prefer to call myself a survivor instead of a victim, but only time will tell if that will hold true. Until then, I'm just going to consider myself a beautiful shade of gray.

What About Family-Focused Intervention?

Catherine A. Marshall

For my father, Algier "Johnny" Marshall, and all of the old, white-haired men and women who slowly came to their feet when James Rogers at the Music Mansion, Pigeon Forge, Tennessee, asked, "Will the veterans please stand?"

As demonstrated in this book, in addition to the supportive and instrumental roles family members can play throughout the cancer experience, family members, as co-survivors, may also face significant stress themselves from a relative's diagnosis of cancer (Baider, Cooper, & Kaplan De-Nour, 2000; Bowman, Rose, & Deimling, 2006; Gustavsson-Lilius, Julkunen, Keskivaara, & Hietanen, 2007; Ferrell, Ervin, Smith, Marek, & Melancon, 2002; Raveis & Pretter, 2005; Sheldon, Ryser, & Krant, 1970; Weihs & Reiss, 2000). Psychologists understand that "cancer appears to be unusually stressful regardless of whether one has it or not. Many people grow up fearing cancer . . ." (Baum & Posluszny, 2001, p. 143). Might it be time to expect family-focused[1] intervention to be available for families facing cancer?

---

[1]The literature also uses the terms family-centered, family-based, and family-oriented interventions with no clear distinction among them. A detailed discussion of the terms family-centered, patient-centered, or patient- and family-centered care, as well as contrasting definitions between family-centered and family-focused, is given at http://www.familycenteredcare.org/faq.html.

While we understand that the family role can be very supportive in cancer treatment and survivorship, as with other chronic illnesses, it is also understood that not all family members are adequately prepared to provide the needed support, especially given that they themselves may well be quite stressed, or not have the needed knowledge or skills, at the time of their relative's cancer diagnosis (Thorne, Bultz, Baile, & The SCRN Communication Team, 2005; Shields & Rousseau, 2004; Woods, Lewis, & Ellison, 1989). Family-based intervention cancer research is needed (Aziz, 2002; Bowman et al., 2006; Kim, Loscalzo, Wellisch, & Spillers, 2006; Northouse, Kershaw, Mood, & Schafenacker, 2005; Mittelman, 2005; Sutherland, Dpsych, White, Jefford, & Hegarty, 2008).

Family-focused intervention does not mean that all family members would be together at all times during any treatment or intervention. For instance, it is understood that family members are not always comfortable sharing their concerns with the relative who has cancer. As reported by Mellon, Berry-Bobovski, Gold, Levin, and Tainsky (2007) in summarizing findings from their focus group research:

> Unaffected relatives talked, sometimes for the first time in the focus groups, about their concerns about loss of their family member and their own fear of getting cancer. However, family members did not feel comfortable in openly discussing these concerns with the cancer survivors, a finding that has also been supported in other research. Tailoring interventions specific to family members is critical to account for their unique anxieties and concerns. Separate educational sessions for family members may be warranted to address their specific worries and questions about risk and how to communicate about risk education within their families. (p. 172)

The Institute for Family-Centered Care provides technical assistance to health organizations to ensure that a family perspective is "reflected in all systems providing care and support to individuals and families including health, education, mental health, and social services" (www.familycenteredcare.org/about/index.html). For instance, the role of the family would be both acknowledged and valued in cancer-related environments. At Dana Farber/Partners CancerCare Program adult oncology program, "patients and families helped revise visiting policies to reflect family-centered principles. As a result, these policies now support and protect patients and recognize the importance of the family's presence, however the patient defines his or her family" (www.familycenteredcare.org/profiles/prof-danafarber.html).

Still, a focus on family is not widespread. Minuchin, Colapinto, and Minuchin (2007) concluded their work with a final chapter, titled "Moving Mountains: Toward a Family Orientation in Service Systems," and delineated the factors needed—at the practitioner, organizational, and societal levels—to support long-term family-focused interventions. Sallis and Owen (2002), in describing ecological models of health behavior, confirmed that "the vast majority of interventions continue to target only the individual level" and that "the difficulty of implementing multilevel approaches should not be underestimated," as "health professionals are usually familiar with individually focused programs but unfamiliar with strategies for policy and environmental change" (p. 469).

Importantly, as demonstrated through several chapters in this book, consideration of culture may often mean consideration of family (Marshall, 2006; Robertson & Flowers, 2007; Marshall, 2008)—another reason why culturally appropriate cancer care, including rehabilitation, would involve consideration of the family. And again, several chapters in this book demonstrate, culture matters in understanding the cancer experience.

Social class is a significant component of culture (Liu et al., 2004) and thus in our work with families facing cancer. Social class is a complex topic—and becomes more complex as it intersects with ethnicity and race. Social class forms essential context for understanding cancer (Freeman, 2004), and yet we too often fail to bring socioeconomic status to the forefront of cancer stories and cancer intervention. Immigrant status is also part of the social class story.

As odd as it may sound, perhaps we need to consider strategies such as that employed by American Indian poet and author Sherman Alexie, who tries his best to attack poverty, illness, any form of pain—with humor and stories. For instance, Alexie (2007), in his autobiographical novel of a poor American Indian boy so determined to obtain an education that he leaves his reservation high school and enrolls in an all-white off-reservation school, describes his two worlds as "White: A Bright Future, Positive Role Models, Hope" and "Indian: A Vanishing Past, A Family History of Diabetes and Cancer, Bone-Crushing Reality" (p. 57). The agenda for this book has been understanding and addressing this "bone-crushing reality" of the cancer experience—how both the person diagnosed with cancer and his or her family as co-survivors are affected.

If not always humor, we have used stories in understanding and addressing cancer. As personal narratives, stories can provide social and emotional context for understanding the intersections of race, ethnicity, gender, and social class in family-focused cancer intervention. As Kreuter et al. (2007) noted, "In large part, the promise and appeal of narrative lies in its familiarity as a basic mode of human interaction. Because people communicate with one another and learn about the world around them largely through stories, it is a comfortable way of giving and receiving information" (p. 222). The stories told in the chapters of this book will hopefully serve, then, to inform not only families who will find them to be excellent and welcomed company in their cancer journey, but also to guide health and human services professionals in finding ways to focus their interventions to include families.

Much work remains in developing systematic and sustainable community-based and community-appropriate intervention for families affected by cancer. A report of the Institute of Medicine (IOM) (Committee on Psychosocial Services, 2007) found that psychosocial interventions in cancer care are "the exception rather than the rule" (p. 1), and recommended that "research address the use of tools and strategies to ensure delivery of appropriate psychosocial services to vulnerable populations, such as those with low literacy, inadequate income, and members of cultural minorities" (pp. 3–4). The IOM report identified six domains of psychosocial problems: (1) Understanding of illness, treatments, and services; (2) Coping with emotions surrounding illness and treatment; (3) Managing illness and health; (4) Behavioral change to minimize disease impact; (5) Managing disruptions in work, school, and family life; and (6) Financial assistance—all consistent with the literature and our experience.

Recent work sponsored by the U.S. National Cancer Institute (Epstein & Street, 2007) calls for "patient-centered communication" while acknowledging the family in the background:

> Patient-centered communication also builds a stronger patient-clinician relationship characterized by mutual trust, respect, and commitment. However, the outcomes of patient-clinician communication must extend beyond the interaction; ideally, communication must also contribute to enhancing the patient's well-being and to reducing suffering after the patient leaves the consultation. For example, a patient-clinician encounter . . . may do little to enhance the patient's well-being if a medical error occurred, if treatment was unacceptably delayed, if access to needed services was not available, or *if subsequent family decisions undermined the intentions and decisions reached in the consultation.* (emphasis added, p. 2)

It remains unclear why family needs, concerns, and decisions would be seen as having "undermined" a process that excluded them. Gustavsson-Lilius et al. (2007) found that female partners of those with cancer displayed more anxiety as well as depression than male partners; at a clinical level, the women's anxiety was higher than that of coronary patients from the authors' previous research. Sutherland and colleagues (2008) found that an Australian cancer education program resulted in "distinct benefits for family and friends," specifically "the adverse effect of living with someone else's cancer may be assuaged through the provision of information, education, and support" (p. 129). These researchers concluded that

> with increasing burden on significant others to provide care to patients, there must be consideration of the needs of this group of people affected by cancer. . . . That family and friends initially reported much lower levels of understanding of cancer and its

treatment along with more negative affect than patients suggests a lack of availability of information and support resources for individuals other than the patient. (p. 131)

Mika Niemelä and Leena Väisänen have described here how a family intervention helps children and young adults understand parental cancer (chapter 4). Might not such an intervention serve all members of the family as well as their service providers? Might not a forward-thinking plan to address the fears and concerns of all affected by a cancer diagnosis prevent the "undermining" of a plan carried out in the relative isolation of a health care provider's office? Why do I care about family-focused cancer intervention? At the conclusion of this book, perhaps it is time to share my story—my father's story—our family story (Marshall, 2008).

Leaving Chattanooga[2]

Leaving Chattanooga, Tennessee, and heading into Georgia, a new sign, complete with a Georgia Peach, designates the narrow two-lane road as officially scenic. The road passes below Lookout Mountain, just below Lover's Leap, where folks do their best to see the Seven States from Rock City. Rock City has barn-sized advertisements all over the South and down I-75, so if you've been in that area, you know what I'm talking about. Chattanooga advertises Rock City as a tourist attraction, but trust me, it's in Georgia.

The postal service told my family when I was growing up that our mailing address was Chattanooga, Tennessee, but, actually, we lived in Georgia. This is the "tri-state area," where mountains, ridges, and hills wind from one state to another and back again. The narrow roads leading to our home in Chattanooga Valley, mostly unmarked when I was a child, now carry street signs. Back then, you had to know where you were going to get there, but now it's easy. From Chattanooga—from St. Elmo, to be specific—take Chattanooga Valley Road (the old road— now the "scenic" road, not the new four-lane highway) to South Avenue, to Mountain View Circle, then at Bluff View Circle, I'm home. This is a beautiful place—"The Valley"—but it is a poor place, a place where ends still don't meet and where people don't go to the doctor until it's too late.

I wrote Daddy's obituary after he died on December 10, 2000. He had been a B-29 gunner. World War II took him away from Southern Appalachia to the North Pacific; I took him to Beacon Hill in Boston, Tucson, and over parts of Australia and Scotland. I wrote in his obituary that he "had resided at the foot of Lookout Mountain in North Georgia, saying that of all his travels he considered Chattanooga Valley and his home to be the most beautiful place in the world." And that's true. He really believed that.

---

[2]Reprinted with permission of the National Rehabilitation Counseling Association.

Daddy was strongly opinionated. I know I get my bull-headedness from him. His name was Algier, but he didn't like that name and told the teachers in school that his name was Johnny. The pastor at his funeral called him "Johnny," as did most folks. Daddy also didn't like grits. I finally asked him just why he didn't like grits so much—I mean, what's not to like about grits? He said it was just that he had eaten so many grits as a kid, as an orphan getting his education at the Berry Schools and working in the kitchen. He said, though, that he'd actually eaten just a lot of cornmeal mush—pretty much the same thing as grits, he said—and demonstrated for me one morning in 2000 just how to make mush—how to be careful to stir the cornmeal slowly into the boiling water.

In her book *Another Country: Navigating the Emotional Terrain of Our Elders*, psychologist Mary Pipher (1999) noted that older persons "don't question their doctors." My family was caught between the old ways of not questioning the doctor's treatment decision and being told that the decisions regarding treatment options rested with us. Physician Rafael Campo (1997) wrote in *The Poetry of Healing: A Doctor's Education in Empathy, Identity, and Desire* that

> to succeed within an HMO, individual patients must indeed become 'health care consumers' more than they can allow themselves to be sick people; the most tirelessly persistent letter writers and phone callers are the ones who obtain timely access not only to providers and referrals to specialists but also to other needed services.

In his copy of Lance Armstrong's (2000) book, *It's Not About the Bike*, Daddy wrote, "See page 93; 98." On page 93, he commented, "Note. This is very important." Armstrong had written about how his treatment had become a "medical collaboration" where he, as the patient, "was as important as the doctor" and where he "began to share the responsibility with them." Physician Jerome Groopman (2000), in his book, *Second Opinions: Stories of Intuition and Choice in the Changing World of Medicine*, wrote that "decisions about diagnosis and treatment are complex. . . . A clinical compass is built not only from the doctor's medical knowledge but also from joining his intuition with that of his patient. . . . It takes time . . . to build trust with a person and to encourage him to express himself." Daddy told me that the most time his oncologist had ever spent with him was about 10 minutes. The researcher in me took over at that point. How could Daddy, how could we as a family, ever make treatment decisions with 10 minutes' worth of information?

On page 98 of Armstrong's book, Daddy marked the words "*What are my chances?* . . . There is no proper way to estimate somebody's chances, and we shouldn't try, because we can never be entirely right, and it deprives people of hope. Hope that is the only antidote to fear." Daddy always seemed to have hope—that's the way he lived his life. Daddy didn't want to die—at all. He wanted to live. In his medical notes, the doctor said that we were both in denial. Yet Daddy did understand that he was dying. He had known for about 48 hours that his cancer was terminal when he said to me, "When you and Ric are home for Christmas, we'll go to the cemetery and pick out a plot. I'm going to be there sooner than I had thought." Daddy died 15 days before Christmas; he didn't have time to pick out his plot, but the folks at the Chattanooga National Cemetery did a fine job. He has a great view of Lookout Mountain—part of those North Georgia mountains that he so loved.

When I left Chattanooga, pretty much for good, after graduation from high school, Daddy took me. He drove me up to Fort Campbell, Kentucky; took me to the office on the army base where I'd spend the summer working for the Screaming Eagles, the 101st Airborne, just back from Vietnam, and then he drove home. He didn't seem particularly alarmed that I didn't have a place to stay; as I recall, he simply left me at a motel. I guess he thought I'd figure it out. Then, in the fall, when I went off to Berry College, Daddy made sure I had my own transportation. He bought an old Pontiac Tempest from the junkyard, an automatic, and installed a "four on the floor." Mechanics always marveled that the car had an automatic transmission lever but also had a four on the floor; what the heck kind of two-in-one transmission was that? After I'd moved out to Arizona, Daddy would always be with Mom at Lovell Field Airport in Chattanooga to pick me up when I came home. Once my nephew was with them and Daddy said, "JT, get me the key for the trunk." Right away, JT opened the back passenger door, picked up a screwdriver from behind the seat, and handed it to Daddy. "Thank you, JT." Daddy opened the trunk and put away my bags. Daddy had a way with cars!

Daddy told me that I'm the first on both sides of my family to graduate from college. He liked to tell jokes, and he liked to tell stories. Once, when I was telling him about how miserable it was to have that Ph.D., to work in academe, but to live on soft money as the research professor who only had the salary that she could bring in through funded grants, he responded, "You know the story about Raggedy Dog, don't you?

So, there was this Raggedy Dog, out in the cold, roaming around, looking for something to eat. Raggedy Dog came upon a good-looking and well-fed dog. This dog had a bowl of food right by the door of his little doghouse and also a bowl of nice clean water—right there. Raggedy Dog said, "Man, you are looking good! And do you have it made, or what?" The good-looking dog responded, "Yes, life is good. My owner brings out fresh food and water for me every day. I'm never hungry. I'm never cold or wet. I've got this great little doghouse right here." Raggedy Dog, said, "Geez, that must be the life! I'd love to have those things." Then Raggedy Dog said, "Hey, what's that thing around your neck?" The good-looking dog responded, "Oh, that's my chain. They keep me chained up and

I can't leave this area except for the little distance the chain allows me to go." Raggedy Dog was quite taken back. He'd never conceived of a life that kept him at chain's length. And it didn't take him long to decide what he wanted to do next. Raggedy Dog went on his way.

Leaving Chattanooga meant going for a higher education. I tended to call home, and Mom and Dad tended to write. I've kept the letters Daddy sent during my education because they kept me going. They are full of love, Daddy's ways, and most of all, they are full of a message that he repeated many times during the years it took me to complete my education—that I could always come home.

Berry College, 1972–1976
August 20, 1975
My Dear,

. . . You know I have told you that our home is your home as long as we have one and you are my little girl and can come home or I'll come get you anytime you want. We haven't had much but what ever we have it's yours. OK. So don't ever put a line on your beautiful brow worrying about that. . . .

The only thing is, you are only going down this road one time and one way—no guarantees or no refunds. I can only hope it will be a joy and gladness. . . . And as far as your life's work, that's what made J. C.'s life what it was—trying to help mankind (or should I say person-kind). Anyway, baby, I love you and you're beautiful . . . Love,

Boston University, Graduate School, 1976–1977
September 11, 1976
My Dear,

It was good to hear from you last nite. Your mom wanted to know why I didn't talk longer. Well to tell the truth, I always try to cut long-distance calls short. Anyway, you sounded well, healthy, and happy so what more should I ask for? After all, that is a lot (an awful lot) for one person to have in one short life time. So why try to improve on that?

Your dog is growing in stature and wisdom. . . . Hope to see you real soon. Love,

October 25, 1976
My Dear!

Yep, at last it's old Dad that takes pen in hand to see what I can pen on some paper on some matters that might be of interest to you.

First off, it has been lonesome without you around the house. Sure miss you. Hope you get home soon, OK. . . .

My dear, I hope you don't make yourself sick by working too hard. Nothing is as important as your health. I can tell you that now because I have been on the road like an old horse.

Here it is time to go again. I'll probably think of a lot of things I should have said. At least here is one I'll say again, "I love you." Take care,

March 20, 1977
My Dear,
   . . . It was good to hear from you the other day and hear your voice. I'll be glad when you do get home. Seems like I'll be old and gone before I find or get time to see you. Strange how fast time goes. Who would think here you are with your Master's Degree. Real proud of you too I might say. I know it has been hard on you and you have had to do without some things but on the other hand you have done a lot and seen a lot you would have otherwise missed! So I do hope the good has been better and outweighed the bad. Must have or you wouldn't have stayed after it like you have. I know the joy of you and your two sisters have been worth all the work and etc that I have gone through so when you plan the rest of your life try not to forget that you too can give the joy of life to some wonderful person like yourself. To have shared my life with you has been great "Thanks."
   . . . Time to go for a walk; hold on. I'll be back in 20 minutes. Well, here I am. This old Bank is a block long and I have to walk it down there and back on 7 floors so that makes it 14 blocks in 20 minutes. Not bad for an old man. Oh yes, I make 7 such trips per nite (98 blocks a nite). . . .
   I know I haven't said much but at least you know we still love you and you still got a place to sleep when you get home. It's yours as long as you want it, OK. . . . Love,

University of Arizona, Doctoral Program, 1980–1984
October 5, 1981
My Dear,
   Thought I'd drop you a note and let you know I'll be there just before the 1st snow fall. "Ha" – Just Kidding. No such luck. Great thought though. . . .
   Old Midnight passed Friday nite. Planted his butt in the backyard. Marked it with an old lawn mower. . . . Take care and I'll see you. Let us know how you are.

February 14, 1982
My Dear,
   Yep, it's your old dad. I'm here at work at that great Temple of Gold, "The American National Bank," in downtown Chattanooga, TN. Not a thing going on so I thought I had better drop my girl a note so as to let her know I'm still kicking and thinking of her. . . . There is only one thing you can do with love to keep it alive and that is to share it. . . .

My Dear: I have told you I don't know the times that as long as I have a home big or small it's your home and you can come home to it anytime for any reason. OK. Hell, hope you do come home. Haven't seen much of you the past years. I almost said few but that wouldn't do. It's been many! Come on home when you want. We love you.

I have been low, low. Haven't missed a day's work but my rear end has drug out all my tracks. Finally went to see a doctor Friday. He didn't know what the hell's wrong but gave me some pills. . . . One thing I will tell you though. Tell [your boyfriend] not to bend over no table should he go see him. Seems they got this gig going. 1st damn time I ever heard of such for a chill but I guess it's something new. . . .

Gota go now. Just wanted you to know we love you. Make sure [your boyfriend] watches those doctors. He'll see why Rover can dish it out but can't take it.

Daddy sure didn't go for those rectal exams. I'm guessing that he successfully avoided another rectal exam "gig" up until the time he was diagnosed with prostate cancer in April 1998 with a PSA of 117.9. That would reflect 16 years of avoidance of the "something new" that might have extended his life. Daddy's constant message of love and the importance of family, the importance of home, and the security that love and family bring is a message that sustains me as I continue to search for my place in academe.

May 9, 1990
My Dear,

Well today your mother and I have been together 42 years. I don't see how she put up with me all these years but she did. You are one of the great products of that 42 years and I'm most proud of you. Even though you have done great things, I know there are greater things to come. I guess I'll have to stick around a while longer to see what they are. By the way, I'm glad your mother has loved me all these years.

Daddy's diagnosis of prostate cancer shook our family. There was the fear of loss, but more importantly, there was the desperate need to understand what prostate cancer was, there was the desperate rush to understand what treatment would be best for Daddy, and there were the desperate attempts to marshal all possible forces to get him to the best possible physician. Through the prostate cancer years, 1998–2000, phone calls, e-mail, and airplanes brought us together. As our family tried to sort out what was going on with treatment, Daddy and I also made our first attempt at playing the stock market!

E-mail, April 9, 2000

Hello, I got your latest note. Must say that bit about the mush was a surprise. Didn't think you would ever try that; glad you did. Sometimes the old ways is the best way. . . . You said a thing about taking kem-0. Please tell the good Dr., I don't give a damn what I have to take or do to get this monkey off my back. Just hope this next test comes up NEGATIVE. Love,

E-mail, October 25, 2000

Hello, Well, we made a few bucks today. . . . I'm just getting the hang of this computer. Anyway, I want to thank you for all you have done for me. Of all the Lepers that Christ healed, only one thanked him. Some deal I'd say. . . . Take care and thanks again.

Medical Records
October 27, 2000

[Patient] is here on a follow-up after he had his implants placed last week. . . . IMPRESSION: Prostate cancer: . . . He did not fill the prescription that I had written the last time. . . . He says he doesn't want to do that now. . . . The cost of these drugs is prohibitive and I can most certainly understand his thoughts on this. . . .

E-mail, November 1, 2000

Hello, This is a day to remember. I have worked all day long. . . . I haven't checked E-Trade today but we made the money yesterday. Oh yes, I forgot to tell you that today is the first day I have felt like working; things are looking better all the time. Love, Dad.

Medical Records
December 1, 2000

[Patient] is here in follow-up of his [bone marrow] biopsy. Unfortunately, the biopsy shows that the bone marrow is packed full of malignant cells, consistent with prostate cancer. IMPRESSION: Metastatic prostate cancer: This is the answer that we have been looking for as to where his metastatic disease is. He has had all the treatments that can be done for his prostate cancer with endocrine manipulation, followed by chemotherapy, and the investigational studies. . . . I think our options are nil, if any. . . . I do not know if he nor his daughter in Arizona are ready to hear this but those are the facts.

December 2, 2000

The patient was discharged home today after a transfusion. . . . He remains at very high risk towards severe bleeding complications. I also spoke with his daughter regarding the event. She has had a lot of problems coming to grips with the reality of what has happened here and it has created some tensions within the family. However, after a long discussion, she seemed to better understand what is going on and recognizes that we appear to be in a terminal situation here.

If I were a songwriter, I'd have the words to a country song; probably that song has already been written and the words are just floating around in my head as memories of music I've danced to. Daddy taught me a lot about living, and he taught me about dying. He taught me about love and the importance of family. He taught me about sticking to work and about leaving before I take too much guff. He taught me about hope and about taking risks—about just going ahead and doing what I needed to do and figuring I'd find a way to pay for it later. And he taught me that I have a home to go back to. It's a place near Chattanooga, at the foot of Lookout Mountain, in a strip of counties that make up the beginnings of Southern Appalachia, and it's a real beautiful place.

References

Alexie, S. (2007). *The absolutely true diary of a part-time Indian*. New York: Little, Brown and Company.

Armstrong, L. (2000). *It's not about the bike: My journey back to life*. New York: G. P. Putnam's Sons.

Aziz, N. M. (2002). Cancer survivorship research: Challenge and opportunity. *International Research Conference on Food, Nutrition, & Cancer*. Conference paper published by the American Society for Nutritional Sciences.

Baider, L., Cooper, C. L., & Kaplan De-Nour, A., (Eds.). (2000). *Cancer and the family* (2nd ed.). New York: John Wiley & Sons.

Baum, A., & Posluszny, D. M. (2001). Traumatic stress as a target for intervention with cancer patients. In A. Baum, & B. L. Andersen, (Eds.), *Psychosocial interventions for cancer* (pp. 143–173). Washington, DC: American Psychological Association.

Bowman, K. F., Rose, J. H., & Deimling, G. T. (2006). Appraisal of the cancer experience by family members and survivors in long-term survivorship. *Psycho-Oncology, 15*(9), 834–845.

Campo, R. (1997). *The poetry of healing: A doctor's education in empathy, identity, and desire*. New York: W. W. Norton & Company.

Committee on Psychosocial Services to Cancer Patients/Families in a Community Setting, Board on Health Care Services. (2007). *Cancer care for the whole patient: Meeting psychosocial health needs*. N. E. Adler & A. E. K. Page (Eds.), Institute of Medicine of The National Academies. Washington, DC: The National Academies Press. http://www.nap.edu/ (Box quote is from "Report Brief, October 2007. For Health Care Providers, p. 4.)

Epstein, R. M., & Street, R. L., Jr. (2007). *Patient-centered communication in cancer care: Promoting healing and reducing suffering*. NIH Publication No. 07–6225. Bethesda, MD: National Cancer Institute.

Ferrell, B., Ervin, K., Smith, S., Marek, T., & Melancon, C. (2002). Family perspectives of ovarian cancer. *Cancer Practice, 10*(6), 269–276.

Freeman, H. P. (2004). Poverty, culture, and social injustice: Determinants of cancer disparities. *CA: A Cancer Journal for Clinicians, 54*, 72–77.

Groopman, J. (2000). *Second Opinions: Stories of intuition and choice in the changing world of medicine.* New York: Viking.

Gustavsson-Lilius, M., Julkunen, J., Keskivaara, P., & Hietanen, P. (2007). Sense of coherence and distress in cancer patients and their partners. *Psycho-Oncology, 16*(12), 1100–1110.

Kim, Y., Loscalzo, M. J., Wellisch, D. K., & Spillers, R. L. (2006). Gender differences in caregiving stress among caregivers of cancer survivors. *Psycho-Oncology, 15*(12), 1086–1092.

Kreuter, M. W., Green, M. C., Cappella, J. N., Slater, M. D., Wise, M. E., Storey, D., et al. (2007). Narrative communication in cancer prevention and control: A framework to guide research and application. *Annals of Behavorial Medicine, 33*(3), 221–235.

Liu, W. M., Ali, S. R., Soleck, G., Hopps, J., Dunston, K., & Pickett, T., Jr. (2004). Using social class in counseling psychology research. *Journal of Counseling Psychology, 51*(1), 3–18.

Marshall, C. A. (2006, March 8). *Ethical practice and cultural factors in rehabilitation: Considering family needs when cancer is the disability.* Training workshop sponsored by the Arizona Rehabilitation Services Administration, Tucson, AZ.

Marshall, C. A. (2008). Family and culture: Using autoethnography to inform rehabilitation practice with cancer survivors. *Journal of Applied Rehabilitation Counseling, 39*(1), 9–19.

Mellon, S., Berry-Bobovski, L., Gold, R., Levin, N., & Tainsky, M. A. (2007). Concerns and recommendations regarding inherited cancer risk: The perspectives of survivors and female relatives. *Journal of Cancer Education, 22*(3), 168–173.

Minuchin, P., Colapinto, J., & Minuchin, S. (2007). *Working with families of the poor* (2nd ed.). New York: Guilford

Mittelman, M. (2005). Taking care of the caregivers. *Current Opinion in Psychiatry, 18*, 633–639.

Northouse, L., Kershaw, T., Mood, D., & Schafenacker, A. (2005). Effects of a family intervention on the quality of life of women with recurrent breast cancer and their family caregivers. *Psycho-Oncology, 14*(6), 478–491.

Pipher, M. (1999). *Another country: Navigating the emotional terrain of our elders.* New York: Riverhead Books.

Raveis, V. H., & Pretter, S. (2005). Existential plight of adult daughters following their mother's breast cancer diagnosis. *Psycho-Oncology, 14*(1), 49–60.

Robertson, S. L., & Flowers, C. R. (2007) Partnering with families for successful career outcomes. In P. Leung, C. R. Flowers, W. B. Talley, & P. R. Sanderson (Eds.), *Multicultural issues in rehabilitation and allied health programs* (pp. 281–301). Linn Creek, MO: Aspen.

Sallis, J. F., & Owen, N. (2002). Ecological models of health behavior. In K. Glanz, B. K. Rimer, F. M. Lewis (Eds.), *Health behavior and health education: Theory, research, and practice* (3rd ed., pp. 462–484). San Francisco: Jossey-Bass.

Sheldon, A., Ryser, C. P., & Krant, M. J. (1970). An integrated family oriented cancer care program: The report of a pilot project in the socio-emotional management of chronic disease. *Journal of Chronic Disease, 22*, 743–755.

Shields, C. G., & Rousseau, S. J. (2004). A pilot study of an intervention for breast cancer survivors and their spouses. *Family Process, 43*(1), 95–107.

Sutherland, G., Dpsych, L. H., White, V. Jefford, M. & Hegarty, S. (2008). How does a cancer education program impact on people with cancer and their family and friends? *Journal of Cancer Education, 23*(2), 126–132.

Thorne, S. E., Bultz, B. D., Baile, W. F., & The SCRN Communication Team. (2005). Is there a cost to poor communication in cancer care? A critical review of the literature. *Psycho-Oncology, 14*(10), 875–884.

Weihs, K., & Reiss, D. (2000). Family reorganization in response to cancer: A developmental perspective. In L. Baider, C. L. Cooper, & A. Kaplan De-Nour (Eds.), *Cancer and the family* (2nd ed., pp. 17–39). New York: John Wiley & Sons.

Woods, N. F., Lewis, F. M., & Ellison, E. S. (1989). Living with cancer: Family experiences. *Cancer Nursing, 12*(1), 28–33.

As mentioned in the introduction to this book, families and co-survivors have told us that they both need information and have been over-whelmed by too much information. Here we list only those resources that we have found to be particularly useful. Chapters in the book also link the reader to specific resources; for instance, chapter 3, "Helping Parents Understand Cancer in Children and Young Adults," provides resources specific to helping a child who is returning to school while recovering from cancer. In chapter 7—"Why Me? Why Anybody?"—disability-related resources are given in the section *What about my job? Can I work?* Chapter 12, "Finding Funds to Help with Cancer Treatment," provides resources for finding financial assistance.

Numerous Web sites are devoted to specific cancers. We suggest that families use one or more of the sites listed here as a starting point for finding information regarding a specific cancer. As Professor Elizabeth Kendall noted in the Foreword, cancer affects families on a worldwide basis. Chapters in this book reflect the international concern with and ex-pertise in cancer. However, the list of resources here is developed from our experience in the United States—we suggest that readers contact their own national and regional cancer societies as well.

National Cancer Organization Web Sites

American Cancer Society

(http://www.cancer.org)
A great place to begin understanding cancer is "Patients, Family, & Friends" at http://www.cancer.org/docroot/home/pff/pff_0.asp. The American Cancer Society provides free brochures on preventing, diag-nosing, and treating different kinds of cancer. Information is available in

hard copy or can be downloaded online. For instance, go to http://
www.cancer.org/asp/freebrochures/fb_global.asp, select "All Categories," and you will see a list of 125 free brochures or booklets, 32 of
which are in Spanish. We appreciate the sentiment behind the title of
one of their resources guides, "Having cancer is hard. Finding help
shouldn't be." A favorite booklet is *After Diagnosis: A Guide for Patients
and Families*; in Spanish, *Después del Diagnóstico: Una Guía para los
Pacientes y sus Familiares.*

CANCERCare

(http://www.cancercare.org)
This national organization has an international reach through its amazing educational workshops conducted via telephone: http://www.
cancercare.org/get_help/tew_calendar.php. CANCER*Care* will call you
at no charge and link you to the workshops—free educational seminars
that address a variety of topics and last one hour. These seminars are
also recorded and archived on their Web site so you can listen to them at
your convenience if you can't make a live call: http://www.cancercare.
org/get_help/tew_faq.php; go to heading "What if I miss a workshop?"
to see a list of workshops that can be heard online. We've selected
just a few favorite and free publications in order to demonstrate their
offerings. Some of their publications are available in Spanish, as well
as other languages such as Russian: http://www.cancercare.org/get_
help/publications.php

(1) *Caregiving for Your Loved One With Cancer*
(2) *Caring Advice for Caregivers: How Can You Help Yourself?*
(3) *Understanding and Managing Chemotherapy Side Effects*
(4) *Doctor, Can We Talk? Tips for Communicating With Your Health Care
Team*
(5) *Helping Children Understand Cancer: Talking to Your Kids About Your
Diagnosis*

Intercultural Cancer Council

(http://iccnetwork.org)
The Intercultural Cancer Council "promotes policies, programs, partnerships, and research to eliminate the unequal burden of cancer among
racial and ethnic minorities and medically underserved populations in
the United States and its associated territories" (http://iccnetwork.org/
who). We appreciate their work and the focus on both our diversity and
our commonalities! Their Cancer Fact Sheets (http://iccnetwork.org/
cancerfacts) are packed with information regarding cancer and racial or
ethnically diverse populations, and also include, for instance, data in
regard to *Rural Poor and the Medically Underserved Americans & Cancer*
and *Workplace & Cancer*, among others.

National Cancer Institute, U.S. National Institutes of Health

(http://www.cancer.gov)
In the United States,

the National Cancer Institute coordinates the National Cancer Program, which conducts and supports research, training, health information dissemination, and other programs with respect to the cause, diagnosis, prevention, and treatment of cancer, rehabilitation from cancer, and the continuing care of cancer patients and the families of cancer patients" (http://www.cancer.gov/aboutnci/overview/mission).

Given this extensive mission, you can expect the National Cancer Institute (NCI) to have extensive and definitive information regarding cancer. Here are just two examples of our favorite publications:

* *Caring for the Caregiver: Support for Cancer Caregivers.*; in Spanish, *Cómo Cuidarse Mientras Usted Cuida a Su Ser Querido: Apoyo para Personas Que Cuidan a un Ser Querido Con Cáncer.*
* *El Equipo de Atención Médica: El Médico es Sólo el Principio* (*Your Health Care Team: Your Doctor Is Only the Beginning*). http://www.cancer. gov/cancertopics/factsheet/rehabilitation/healthcare-team-spanish. (We've only been able to find this information in Spanish—English or other language speakers, ask NCI if they can provide a translation for you. We like this publication because it explains the role of cancer team members and includes professionals involved in rehabilitation.)

National Coalition for Cancer Survivorship

(http://www.canceradvocacy.org)
The National Coalition for Cancer Survivorship is "the oldest survivor-led cancer advocacy organization in the country" (http://www. canceradvocacy.org/about), and we like their resources listed at http:// www.canceradvocacy.org/resources. For instance, we recommended in chapter 7 the publication *Working It Out: Your Employment Rights As A Cancer Survivor.*

Tackling the Stresses of the Cancer Experience

Most likely you have your own ideas about how to reduce your stress—maybe it's gardening, maybe it's yoga—have you tried laughter yoga? If not, perhaps you can find an instructor near you—there are classes, for instance, at the Benson-Henry Institute for Mind Body Medicine (http:// www.massgeneral.org/bhi/services/treatmentprograms.aspx?id=1316). Located at Massachusetts General Hospital in Boston, the Benson-Henry Institute reports that 60–90% of all visits to a physician are for conditions related to stress. Mind-body interactions are defined as relaxation response, nutrition, exercise, and spirituality (http://www.massgeneral.org/bhi/about). It is exciting to see what once was "alternative" now considered "integrative," so we start there in regard to offering favorite resources for dealing with stress.

Integrative Medicine (also referred to as Integrative Oncology)

The Integrative Medicine Service at Memorial Sloan-Kettering Cancer Center "was established in 1999 to complement mainstream medical care and address the emotional, social, and spiritual needs of patients and families" (http://www.mskcc.org/mskcc/html/1979.cfm). This Web site links to information about therapies that can help deal with the stress of cancer, for instance: **aromatherapy, massage, reflexology, reiki, meditation, acupuncture, qi gong, yoga**, and more. As one example, for more about acupuncture, see Sloan-Kettering's description of the benefits of this "form of traditional Chinese medicine" at http://www.mskcc.org/mskcc/html/1987.cfm#4.

Acutonics®

Remember that in dealing with stress there are always alternatives—and there are always alternatives to the alternatives! If improved energy sounds good, but perhaps not needles, even ultra-thin ones, acutonics can provide an alternative. Defined in part as "the application of tuning forks . . . to acupuncture points," acutonics allows "noninvasive access into these core energetic systems within the body" (http://www.acutonics.com). For more information about acutonics or sound acupuncture, see http://www.optimumhealthandbeyond.com/sound_healing.html.

Exercise

Whether walking, jogging, running, or swimming, for instance, exercise is understood to be both beneficial for the body and a stress reliever. The National Center on Physical Activity and Disability, "an information center concerned with physical activity and disability" (http://www.ncpad.org), provides specific information regarding the benefits of exercise in an online article titled "Disability/Condition: Cancer and Exercise" (http://www.ncpad.org/disability/fact_sheet.php?sheet=195).

Expressive Arts

The expressive arts "combine the visual arts, movement, drama, music, writing and other creative processes to foster deep personal growth and community development" (http://www.ieata.org/about.html). You may have recognized the therapeutic aspects of listening to or playing music, drawing, etc., but if you'd like further ideas on ways the arts can help reduce the stress of a cancer journey, check out cancer center Web sites for their expressive arts programs. For instance, the Cancer Therapy & Research Center at The University of Texas Health Science at San

Antonio offers classes in making a scrapbook and journaling (http://www.ctrc.net/ctrc_2_2.cfm?db_content=calart).

Further Information

Several chapters in this book provide references that can be used for obtaining further information. Countless Web sites can link you to the latest information regarding cancer, survivorship, and the concerns families face. We conclude with two favorites:

* If you want access to recent technical and medical information regarding cancer, try http://www.cancernetwork.com, which provides free access to the medical journal *ONCOLOGY* as well as a partner publication, *Oncology NEWS International.*
* National Comprehensive Cancer Network (NCCN) is an alliance of cancer centers (http://www.nccn.org/members/network.asp) that develops clinical practice guidelines in oncology. "Although the NCCN Clinical Practice Guidelines in Oncology™ are written for physicians and other healthcare professionals, anyone may access these professional guidelines free of charge" (http://www.nccn.com/AboutUs/Default.aspx?id=73). Stating that "knowledge is power in the fight against cancer," the NCCN has also developed a user-friendly "consumer" Web site (http://www.nccn.com) that provides a summary of the clinical practice guidelines.

About the Editor and Contributors

THE EDITOR

Catherine A. Marshall, Ph.D., CRC, NCC, is research professor in the Department of Educational Psychology, Northern Arizona University. She is Frances McClelland Associate Research Professor; Frances McClelland Institute for Children, Youth, & Families; Norton School of Family & Consumer Sciences at the University of Arizona (UA). She is a senior scholar with the UA National Center of Excellence in Women's Health and an adjunct professor, Centre for National Research on Disability and Rehabilitation Medicine, Griffith University, Australia. In 2007, Catherine received a two-year Ruth L. Kirschstein National Research Service Award for Individual Senior Fellowship, funded by the Department of Health and Human Services, National Institutes of Health, National Cancer Institute to support her work regarding the impact of the cancer experience on the family. Catherine has more than 30 years of experience working in the field of rehabilitation. In 1997, she received the National Council on Rehabilitation Education Outstanding Researcher of the Year award for research with American Indian families and chronic illness/ disability. As a Fulbright scholar, she researched the needs and resources of indigenous people with disabilities in Oaxaca, Mexico. Catherine is founder and president of the nonprofit organization Women's International Leadership Institute (www.wili.org), which benefits low-income women seeking to improve their educational and economic status.

THE CONTRIBUTORS

Alice F. Chang, Ph.D., was diagnosed with breast cancer in 1993. She went on to found the Academy for Cancer Wellness, a nonprofit organization in Tucson, Arizona, that recognizes the courage of cancer survivors and their families, supports research into living with cancer, and provides bridge funding for underinsured cancer patients. Alice is the author of *A Survivor's Guide to Breast Cancer* (New Harbinger Press, 2000). She received her undergraduate degree from UCLA in 1968 and her Ph.D. from University of Southern California in 1973. In addition to serving on many governance boards of local, regional, and national organizations, she has received Distinguished Contributions awards from the American Psychological Association (APA) and the UCLA Alumni Award of Excellence in Public Service.

Alice was the first ethnic minority woman to be elected to the APA Board of Directors. Her clinical practice involves disseminating and promoting the understanding of coping mechanisms associated with adjustment among those who have been touched by cancer and other chronic illnesses. In addition, she addresses identity and behavioral issues related to gender and/or ethnicity, particularly among Asian Americans and Pacific Islander populations.

Mark Clark has been employed in law enforcement for more than 37 years and resides in Queensland, Australia. Married with two grown children and two grandchildren, he has found time to obtain master's degrees in public policy and administration (Charles Sturt), a Bachelor of Science (sociology, Excelsior College), and a professional Diploma of Corporate Management (Institute of Corporate Managers, Chartered Secretaries & Administrators). He is now enrolled in a Ph.D. program at Bond University. His interests include reading, exercise, watching sports, and a renewed interest in travel.

Joyce A. DeVoss, Ph.D., is an associate professor in the Department of Educational Psychology at Northern Arizona University. She is currently coordinator of the M.Ed. School Counseling Program at Northern Arizona University in Tucson and co-chair of the Arizona School Counseling Association (AzSCA) Research Committee. She teaches courses in counseling theory, counseling processes, group processes, marriage and family counseling, child and adolescent counseling, and practicum and internship. She is the first author of a book titled *School Counselors as Educational Leaders* (2006), and also has written articles and book chapters on school-counseling related topics. She has presented her work at local, state, national, and international levels. She is a licensed psychologist and has treated children and families with loved ones who were cancer patients.

Deirdre Cobb-Roberts, Ph.D., is associate professor of social foundations in the Department of Psychological and Social Foundations at the University of South Florida and a former McKnight Junior Faculty Fellow. Deirdre teaches graduate courses in multicultural education and history of American higher education. Her research has focused on the history of American higher education and teacher education with an emphasis on cultural diversity. She is particularly interested in the benefits of historical examination of diversity; how students, faculty, and institutions respond to diversity in colleges and universities; and pre-service teachers' resistance to diversity.

Paul Donnelly's work has received 26 full productions and numerous readings at venues in Washington, DC; Normal, Illinois; Cleveland and

Cincinnati, Ohio; Asheville, North Carolina; Memphis, Tennessee; and Charlottesville and Richmond, Virginia. His work won the Larry Neal Writers Award for Drama (DC Commission on the Arts and Humanities), the Virginia Playwriting Fellowship (Virginia Commission for the Arts), and first and third prizes in the Source Theatre Company National Ten-Minute Playwriting Contest. He was twice nominated for Washington, DC's, Helen Hayes Award for Outstanding New Play. He has directed nine full productions, including five world premieres and one English-language premiere. Paul was pleased to serve six times as playwright-in-residence for New Voices for the Stage, a program that brings high school playwrights from across the state of Virginia to Richmond for three weeks of classes with theater professionals and collaboration in developing workshop productions. Paul has also taught playwriting at St. Mary's College of Maryland, the Writer's Center in Bethesda, Maryland, and Theatre Lab in Washington, DC.

Maria C. Figueroa is a program coordinator at the College of Nursing, University of Arizona, and currently recruits patients for two breast cancer studies and a prostate cancer study that explore the effectiveness of psychosocial and/or educational counseling via telephone. This work allows Maria the opportunity to meet not only people struggling with cancer but also their families. In particular, Maria appreciates the opportunity to educate Latinas about breast cancer, as well as connect them with services in the community as needed. Maria also has worked at the Arizona Cancer Center, where she worked closely with patients diagnosed with cancer and their families to ensure they had access to treatment and assistance, both financial and emotional.

Alma E. Flores, MSW, LCSW, is a clinical social worker with more than 20 years of postgraduate experience working in the public health sector, specializing in the treatment of patients with chronic illnesses such as mental health, HIV/AIDS, and cancer. Alma is professionally trained as a bilingual/bicultural social worker. Her work and advocacy efforts have addressed the needs of underserved Latinos and other less privileged populations in the states of New Jersey and Florida. Inspired by personal losses to cancer, in 2004 she cofounded LUNA (*Latinos Unidos por un Nuevo Amanecer* [Latinos United for a New Awakening]) de Pinellas, a support group for Latino cancer survivors and their loved ones. Alma works as a counselor, support group facilitator, and cancer care navigator at CaPSS (Cancer Patient Support Services Program), Bay Care-Morton Plant Mease Health Care in Clearwater, Florida. She has held volunteer affiliation with and served on the LUNA, Inc. Executive Board since 2005.

Lena R. Gaddis, Ph.D., is an associate professor in the Department of Educational Psychology at Northern Arizona University. Her professional expertise as a school psychologist is in working with children and adolescents with disabilities and their families. Lena's research expertise is in cognitive and social/affective development of children and adolescents, with a special interest on the educational needs of child survivors of cancer.

Rose Gordon is a graduate of Indiana University South Bend and holds her Master of Ministries degree from Bethel College in Mishawaka, Indiana. She works as a staff nurse for the North Carolina Department of Corrections and is a volunteer hospital chaplain. Rose is the author of two short stories, "The Rainbow" (2000) and "The Tree Swing" (2001), both in *Heartwarmers*. She is a member of P.E.O. chapter CG sisterhood, an educational philanthropic organization. She lives in the Blue Ridge Mountains with her husband, John, and their four dogs, Sammy, Kirby, Spikey, and Molly Muffin.

Sharon R. Johnson, MS, CRC, a consultant in participatory research and cancer, is retired from the State of Minnesota, Division of Rehabilitation Services, after more than 30 years as a rehabilitation counselor. During that time, she provided services to American Indians living on reservations in northern Minnesota. Sharon is an enrolled member of the Minnesota Chippewa Tribe and worked to develop culturally appropriate service delivery to American Indians with disabilities through the public vocational rehabilitation program. A breast cancer survivor and the mother of a cancer survivor, in 2002 she completed a cancer research training fellowship through the Native Researchers Cancer Control Training Program, Oregon Health & Science University and University of Arizona. Sharon has authored or co-authored several professional publications that are derived from her involvement in community-based, participatory action research involving people with disabilities and cancer.

Lorraine Johnston is the wife of a 19-year lymphoma survivor and the daughter of a more than 35 years lymphoma survivor. In the years since her husband's diagnosis, she has been involved in a number of support groups that offer emotional and practical support to lymphoma survivors. Her first book was *Non-Hodgkin's Lymphomas: Making Sense of Diagnosis, Treatment & Options*. In the course of her support group efforts, Lorraine has been interviewed by the *Philadelphia Inquirer* and by National Public Radio's *Marketplace* program regarding the best ways to find reliable medical information using a personal computer and various media such as the World Wide Web. She attempts to dispel the myths that access to sound medical information is cloaked in secrecy and that medical literature is impossible to interpret. Using her lifelong love of biology and her degree in life sciences, she helps cancer survivors evaluate accurately the material they locate, emphasizing resources such as the National Cancer Institute's databases of treatments and clinical trials, and the National Library of Medicine's MEDLINE. Lorraine's years of study have included many courses in psychology, but she found that nothing in her educational background prepared her adequately for facing the terror and heartbreak of cancer. One of her chief interests is helping the newly diagnosed as well as long-term survivors feel less lonely and less afraid as they confront their diagnoses and weigh their options.

Claudia X. Aguado Loi, MPH, is earning her Ph.D. in health education and behavioral health at the University of South Florida. She is trained as an epidemiologist and in using mixed methodology research design and analysis. Her area of expertise is cancer health disparities. Claudia has been instrumental in seeking funding for and coordinating many multimillion-dollar studies funded by the National Institutes of Health and the Centers for Disease Control, addressing, for instance, Latino health disparities, mild depression, and cancer prevention and control. Most recently, she has become involved in community-based participatory research addressing mental health. Claudia's local community commitment is reflected by her involvement and volunteer service to LUNA, Inc. (*Latinos Unidos por un Nuevo Amanecer* [Latinos United for a New Awakening]), beginning in 2004. She is a member of the Tampa Bay Community Cancer Network. Cancer has personally affected her immediate family, close friends, and fellow colleagues. Their experiences have inspired her to continue her volunteer work with LUNA, to work in the oncology field, and to contribute to the collaborative effort of this volume.

Anne Mallett, MSW, LISW/LCSW, is a social worker with over 13 years of social service experience in a variety of settings, including hospital, residential, group home, and corrections. Anne is currently an outpatient therapist, providing individual, family, and couples counseling at a non-profit organization as well as in private practice. Anne is a Medical Reserve Corp volunteer and a board member for Mothers & More Defiance Chapter.

Mika Niemelä, MHSc, is project manager for the nationwide Effective Child & Family program, administered through Finland's National Institute for Health and Welfare. The Effective Child & Family program develops preventative and health promoting services for children and families when a parent has difficulties such as psychiatric problems or drug abuse. Mika has worked as a family therapist and family therapy trainer at Oulu University Hospital, Oulu, Finland. He is a specialist in family interventions when a parent has cancer.

Rebecca Paradies is an artist and a horse enthusiast. She holds a master's degree in expressive arts therapy from the European Graduate School in Saas-Fee, Switzerland, and an undergraduate degree in studio art from the University of Arizona. She paints from her experiences of travels around the world and includes her own horses and those she knows (www.paintinghorses.net). Rebecca has nine years of experience working therapeutically in the expressive arts field and has focused during the last seven years on combining the equine experience and deepening this experience through the expressive arts. Rebecca maintains a private practice in Tucson, Arizona, and also works on a locked psychiatric unit, providing expressive arts therapy to those who have been deemed a danger to themselves or others.

Monica R. Robinson is a native of Tucson, Arizona. She is a wife to Bradford Robinson and mother to Jessica and Krystin Robinson. Monica loves spending quality time with her husband; together, they support their daughters' interests in basketball and dance. After living in Georgia for 10 years, Monica and Bradford returned to Arizona in order to raise their girls surrounded by family. Monica enjoys reading and movies, currently works in community health, and hopes to return to school for a degree in nursing.

Ilkka Saarnio is a lymphoma survivor and a prostate cancer survivor. He is involved in the patient support activities of the Pirkanmaa Cancer Association (PCA), a regional organization of the Cancer Society of Finland. Through the PCA, Ilkka provides peer support to individuals diagnosed with cancer and also conducts peer group discussions. His professional background is in research and development of medical and assistive technology.

Sarah Sample, MSW, RSW, is a social worker at the British Columbia Cancer Agency in Vancouver, where she has worked for 18 years in the Patient and Family Counseling Services program, providing individual, family, and group counseling. Sarah previously taught in the School of Social Work at the University of British Columbia, Canada. Her particular interests include the impact on families facing cancer and coping with anxiety. Her other main areas of interest are complementary therapies for patients and their families living with cancer, which include mindfulness-based stress reduction, therapeutic touch, and guided visualization. Since 1998, Sarah facilitates the first and only lesbian and bisexual support group in a Canadian cancer treatment center.

Gloria I. San Miguel, MSHS, is a health care executive with more than seven years of postgraduate experience in the operations management of hospitals. She is currently responsible for the management and quality process improvement of clinical and nonclinical areas, including the Cancer Patient Support Services Program for Oncology at Morton Plant Mease Health Care in Clearwater, Florida. Gloria has 10 years of clinical trials and academic research experience. Her personal losses to cancer and her daily experiences as a manager of cancer services have motivated her to use her leadership role to eliminate service provision barriers for underserved cancer patients. Her grant writing expertise has been fundamental in obtaining funding for Camp Alegria and for the development and sustainability of free cancer prevention and patient service programs. Gloria's commitment to eliminating cancer care disparities is evidenced by her many professional and civic affiliations: executive board member, Pinellas Suncoast region of the American Cancer Society; Tampa Bay Community Cancer Network (TBCCN), Moffitt Cancer Center and Research Institute Steering committee member; executive board member, LUNA, Inc. (*Latinos Unidos por un Nuevo Amanecer* [Latinos United for a New Awakening]); American College of Healthcare Executives (ACHE), Western Florida Chapter, board member/ director-at-large since 2004; and board member of "La Clinica Guadalupana," a free clinic, mostly for Latinos, in Clearwater, Florida.

Dinorah (Dina) Martinez Tyson, Ph.D., MPH, is bilingual (English/ Spanish) and is academically trained in applied medical anthropology and epidemiology. She is an assistant research professor in the College of Behavioral and Community Sciences, Department of Aging and Mental Health Disparities at the University of South Florida. She has extensive experience in community-based participatory research, and has worked closely with various Latino community organizations to address health disparities. Dr. Martinez Tyson worked at H.T. Lee Moffitt Cancer Institute, a comprehensive cancer research center and hospital, from 2001 to 2008. One of her main roles there was to adapt cultural and linguistically relevant psychosocial interventions for Latinos. She has made fundamental contributions to LUNA (*Latinos Unidos por un Nuevo Amanecer* [Latinos United for a New Awakening]) since she became a volunteer for the original group in 2003. Dr. Martinez Tyson led the organization's incorporation process; coordinates Camp Alegria, LUNA's signature event; founded a LUNA Tampa support group in 2005; and continues to facilitate the group on a monthly basis.

Leena Väisänen, MD, Ph.D., is a psychiatrist at Oulu University Hospital, Oulu, Finland. A psychiatric consultant in health centers as well, she is a specialist in family therapy and family medicine. Leena is also a trainer and supervisor for The Effective Family project in Finland and has supervised family interventions in families with parental cancer.

About the Series Editors and Board of Advisors

THE SERIES EDITORS

Catherine A. Marshall, Ph.D., CRC, NCC, is research professor in the Department of Educational Psychology, Northern Arizona University. She is Frances McClelland Associate Research Professor; Frances McClelland Institute for Children, Youth, & Families; Norton School of Family & Consumer Sciences at the University of Arizona (UA). She is a senior scholar with the UA National Center of Excellence in Women's Health and an adjunct professor, Centre for National Research on Disability and Rehabilitation Medicine, Griffith University, Australia. In 2007, Catherine received a two-year Ruth L. Kirschstein National Research Service Award for Individual Senior Fellowship, funded by the Department of Health and Human Services, National Institutes of Health, National Cancer Institute to support her work regarding the impact of the cancer experience on the family. Catherine has more than 30 years of experience working in the field of rehabilitation. In 1997, she received the National Council on Rehabilitation Education Outstanding Researcher of the Year award for research with American Indian families and chronic illness/disability. As a Fulbright scholar, she researched the needs and resources of indigenous people with disabilities in Oaxaca, Mexico. Catherine is founder and president of the nonprofit organization Women's International Leadership Institute (www.wili.org), which benefits low-income women seeking to improve their educational and economic status.

Elizabeth Kendall, Ph.D., is a research professor at the Griffith Institute of Health and Medical Research, Griffith University, and associate director of the Centre for National Research on Disability and Rehabilitation, at Griffith University and University of Queensland. She holds a Bachelor of Arts in psychology and special education and postgraduate qualifications in rehabilitation psychology. Elizabeth completed her doctorate in 1997 on adjustment following traumatic brain injury and received the Dean's Commendation for Outstanding Ph.D. Thesis (University of Queensland). She was awarded a Medal for Excellence in Research Supervision in 1999, and all her graduate students have also received commendations for excellence. For the past 20 years, she has maintained both a community/clinical practice and a research agenda in the issues faced by people with acquired disabilities or chronic conditions. She has focused on participatory methods for developing innovative service models. Elizabeth has published in more than 60 international peer-reviewed journals and books and maintains an active role in the development of nongovernment organizations that address gaps in service delivery for people with disability or chronic disease. She is a series co-editor of *Disability Insights and Issues*, published by Praeger.

THE BOARD OF ADVISORS

Martha E. Banks, Ph.D., received her A.B. in psychology from Brown University and completed her training in the American Psychological Association (APA)-approved Clinical Psychology Program at the University of Rhode Island, followed by an APA-approved internship at the Des Moines Child Guidance Center. She is an APA fellow and a fellow of the Society for Women in Psychology. Martha is a former member of the APA Council and former president of the Society for the Psychology of Women. Her service to APA was recognized with a presidential citation in 2008. Martha has also been a professor of Black Studies at The College of Wooster. She has more than 30 years of professional experience as a clinician, researcher, and professor in psychology. Martha co-edited the book set *Disability: Insights from Across Fields and Around the World* and the book *Women with Visible and Invisible Disabilities: Multiple Intersections, Multiple Issues, Multiple Therapies*. Martha has been involved with the neuropsychological assessment and treatment of female victims of abuse and conducts ongoing research involving the Ackerman-Banks Neuropsychological Rehabilitation Battery.

Lesley Chenoweth, Ph.D., is the inaugural professor of social work and codirector of the Griffith Institute of Health and Medical Research at Griffith University in Australia. She has more than 35 years of experience as a social work and human service practitioner and academic, 20 of these in the disability area. Lesley's research has spanned disability issues, human services, rural communities, welfare reform, recruitment and retention in human service organizations, child welfare, social work practice, disability policy analysis, deinstitutionalization, families, violence, and abuse. She is a consultant to government and community organizations and has served on numerous boards and committees for disability, legal, and family welfare agencies. Lesley serves on several editorial boards and is a regularly invited speaker in Australia and overseas.

Sharon R. Johnson, MS, CRC, a consultant in participatory research and cancer, is retired from the State of Minnesota, Division of Rehabilitation Services, after more than 30 years as a rehabilitation counselor. During that time she provided services to American Indians living on reservations in northern Minnesota. Sharon is an enrolled member of the Minnesota Chippewa Tribe and worked to develop culturally appropriate service delivery to American Indians with disabilities through the public vocational rehabilitation program. A breast cancer survivor and the mother of a cancer survivor, in 2002 she completed a cancer research training fellowship through the Native Researchers Cancer Control Training Program, Oregon Health & Science University and University of Arizona. Sharon has authored or co-authored several professional publications that are derived from her involvement in community-based, participatory action research involving people with disabilities and cancer.

Paul Leung, Ph.D., is a professor in the Department of Rehabilitation, Social Work and Addictions at the University of North Texas. He has held previous academic and administrative appointments at Deakin University (Melbourne, Australia), the University of Illinois–Urbana, the University of North Carolina at Chapel Hill, and the University of Arizona. Paul's interests have included rehabilitation and disability of persons from diverse racial/ethnic backgrounds and students with disabilities. He is a fellow of the American Psychological Association (APA) and a past president of APA's Division of Rehabilitation Psychology (22), the National Council on Rehabilitation Education, and the National Association of Multicultural Rehabilitation Concerns. He is a recipient of APA's Division 22 Lifetime Achievement Award.